DRUGS FOR LESS

DRUGS FOR LESS

*The Complete Guide to Free
and Discounted Prescription Drugs*

*Featuring More Than 600 of the Most
Commonly Prescribed Medications*

MICHAEL P. CECIL, M.D.

FOREWORD BY FERROL SAMS, JR., M.D.

healthyliving**books**

New York • London

A Healthy Living Book
Published by Hatherleigh Press
5-22 46th Avenue, Suite 200
Long Island City, NY 11101
www.hatherleighpress.com

Library of Congress Cataloging-in-Publication Data

Cecil, Michael P.
 Drugs for less : the complete guide to free and discounted prescription
drugs, featuring more than 600 of the most commonly prescribed medications / Michael
P. Cecil.
    p. cm.
 "A Healthy Living Book."
 ISBN 1-57826-192-9
 1. Drugs--Popular works. 2. Generic drugs--Popular works. 3.
Drugs--Costs--Popular works. I. Title.
 RM301.15.C43 2005
 615'.1--dc22

                        2005001937

Drugs for Less is available for bulk purchase, special promotions, and premiums. For information on reselling and special purchase opportunities, call 1-800-528-2550 and ask for the Special Sales Manager.

Interior design by Eugenie Delaney and Deborah Miller
Cover design by Deborah Miller and Phillip Mondestin

10 9 8 7 6 5 4 3 2 1
Printed in Canada

TO SUDI

Acknowledgments

BEING A CARDIOLOGIST gives me a front-row seat on the stage of life with its wide diversity. I have cared for generals, politicians, CEOs, prisoners, and many extraordinary people living what they believe are ordinary lives. Patients have confided their concerns, and many have touched me deeply. In recent years, my office staff have been greatly moved by our patients' predicament of being unable to afford their medications. Modern drugs may be lifesaving, but only for those fortunate enough to afford them.

I went to the bookstore to look for a book discussing how people could obtain their medications at a reduced cost. When I couldn't find a book, I decided to write *Drugs for Less*—but I needed a great deal of help. My office staff helped me to compile long lists of pharmaceutical assistance programs and gleaned additional information from pharmaceutical representatives. Pharmacists taught me which pills can be safely sliced into two parts, which medications have generic substitutes, and how medications are priced. Resourceful patients shared the novel methods they use to lower their cost.

I was well supported by family, friends, and colleagues, who encouraged me during the process. Many friends and colleagues donated large amounts of their time to improve the manuscript including Amy Byrd, Susie Cassarino, Dr. Robert Halliday, Dr. Mark Hanson, Dr. Royce Hanson, Dr. Steve Macheers, Dr. Andrew Malinchak, Mark Moscip, Kristen Patton, Dr. Alan Perreiah, and Dr. Warren Schultz. I am grateful that my literary agent, Dan Bial, introduced me to my skillful editor, Andrea Au, and enthusiastic publisher, Hatherleigh Press.

Finally, and most important, my deepest thanks go to my wife, Sudi. Without her inspiration and love, I could not have written this book.

Foreword

OLD FOLKS WORRY. They should. The grasshopper has not sung its September song into a cheerful and early demise but has been transmogrified into the frantic ant, which scurries incessantly to store up food for the winter.

Humans plan ahead for the predeath experience called retirement. Their working years are rhythmically and habitually devoted to setting aside money so that they can quit working and enjoy their declining years in leisure and comfort. I call retirement the holding pond.

I do not think they necessarily worry about dying itself. Mr. Dean Murphy, an acerbic and opinionated octogenarian, said to me, "Sambo, somebody asked me the other day, 'Who in the hell wants to live to be ninety years old?' and I looked him in the eye and said, 'Any sum-bitch who is eighty-nine!'"

Miss Louise Murphy, Mr. Dean's widow, at age 90, listened to her daughter say that it was about time to cash in one of her CDs and replied, "We'll do no such thing; Dean left me those for my old age."

She had analyzed worry for me years before: "When you get old and have a long tail of children and grandchildren strung out behind you, all of them start trying to 'protect' you. They won't discuss things they think will upset you. They don't realize that you have already lived through more trials and worries than all of them combined, nor does it enter their heads that we can always tell when they are concealing something from us. Now, that's where real worry comes in—they don't understand that when we know they're hiding something, we automatically start imagining what can be wrong, and the reality is never as bad as what we imagine.

"When I was lying in the hospital after my operation, a delegation came piling into my room at visiting hours, a whole gaggle of them, and they chattered and nattered about this, that, and the other, and not a one of them would make eye contact with me. I knew something was wrong, and when they finally cleared out I lay there in a state, worrying about everything under the shining sun.

"They hadn't been gone twenty minutes before my phone rang, and it was my daughter-in-law, good ol' Boots, who will always tell her guts, you know, and she said, 'What do we do when our friends the Stells die?' And I said, 'We get in the kitchen and cook! Which one was it?'"

I don't think old people worry about dying nearly as much as the middle-aged group. Most of the elderly have executed wills and put them safely in a drawer (and thus out of mind). They then devote their energies to the demands of daily living.

Miss Louise anticipated death with equanimity. "Ferrol, I had hoped the good Lord was going to spare me from going through another Christmas, but here it is upon us so I guess I'll have to smile and endure another one."

Instead, old people worry about money. The term "fixed income" has become a shibboleth among them, has become almost a denigrating definition of Social Security, pensions, and Medicare.

Miss Louise anticipated this years before Mr. Dean died. "Dean, I do hope with all the things you are doing in that high-faluting law firm in Atlanta that you are arranging things so that I won't have to go and live with any of the children or grandchildren when you die!"

Mr. Dean, ever the pragmatist, replied in consolation, "Louise, I have left you pretty well fixed. If you just don't live too damn long."

Long before Lyndon Johnson broke loose out of Texas, Miss Lou Jones, a salty nonagenarian, told me, "When my husband died, and I'll tell you straight out I looked at him in the casket and said, 'Well, at least now I know where you are every night.' He left me pretty well fixed. Comfortable, you might say; not rich. But the trouble is I've outlived my income: I'm too blasted old."

Nowadays I hear patients say, "I can't afford that medicine; I'm on a fixed income, you know."

"Fixed," of course, beats "no" income, but we're talking here about the elderly, and this is what I hear them worrying about. They don't want to have strokes, heart attacks, end-stage renal disease, uncontrolled diabetes, or to have to live with their children, each of which events would be a disastrous disruption of their lives; but the economic reality is that a large number of them are truly in a bind.

Equally in a bind are a great number of younger people. So many of them are working for minimum wage or else have young children and no health insurance. As long as they are not paying $3.00 a day for cigarettes, my heart goes out to them also. How can we help them?

Enter Mike Cecil.

Michael Cecil is, of a certainty, no ordinary man, and he is a most extraordinary physician. Beyond his chosen specialty of cardiology, he maintains a keen interest in all aspects of medicine. Paramount among his virtues is a genuine concern for each individual patient; he knows each one of them; he knows their backgrounds, their family problems, their financial worries.

From the interconnection with his fellow humans, and in the midst of a voluminous daily roll of patients, somehow this man has found the time to research and prepare the information in this book. Carefully perused, it should save the sick folk of America a considerable amount of money.

If physicians would use it as a guide for their prescribing habits, they could render a service beyond the science of medicine. Material considerations should ever be one facet of the art of medicine.

This book is a tribute to the love and concern of one practicing physician for the elderly and the poor. Beneath its matter-of-fact detailing of prices and comparable analyses of various drugs lies the dedication and determination of a very spiritual Doctor of Medicine. I recommend this book to everyone.

—*Ferrol Sams, Jr., M.D.*

Dr. Ferrol Sams, Jr. is the author of seven novels, including *Run with the Horseman,* and he is recognized as one of Georgia's finest authors. Mercer University established the Ferrol A. Sams, Jr., Distinguished Chair of English in 1994. Now an active octogenarian, Dr. Sams practices medicine in Fayette County full-time, as he has done for more than fifty years.

Disclaimer

This book is for informational and educational purposes only, and it is not a substitute for the professional medical or legal advice given to you by your attorney, your physician, and or any other professional advisers.

Using this book should not substitute for the advice of your physician and does not create a doctor-patient relationship. You are strongly advised to follow the advice of your physician, pharmacists, and other health care providers who know the specifics of your medical condition. Do not use any information in this book without first consulting your health care providers.

The patients and characters in the book are based on real patients, but the names and details have been changed.

Contents

Preface

THE NUMBER OF MY PATIENTS who cannot afford their prescription drugs has grown dramatically during the past few years. Medications greatly enhance health and quality of life; however, they are beneficial only to those who can pay for them. As a cardiologist, I primarily see patients with heart disease, whose inability to buy prescription drugs can be lethal. For some, it comes down to a choice between buying medications and buying food.

My office staff and I have been touched by this mounting problem, and we have tried to respond. Our search of magazines, books, websites, and discussion groups for information on reducing prescription drug costs came to one conclusion: such information is surprisingly difficult to find. The problem of rising drug prices is widely reported in newspapers and on television, but practical solutions are seldom given. So we did a little more research.

Patients told us about pharmacies with the best prices, as well as novel methods of purchasing medications from Canada and Indian tribes. Pharmacists taught us which drugs can be purchased as low-cost generic substitutes and which medications can be safely divided, or "sliced." Pharmaceutical representatives were generous in supplying drug samples and offered information regarding pharmaceutical assistance programs.

This guidebook is the result of our work. We discovered that a wealth of information exists on how to reduce prescription drug costs, but this information is not well known to the general public. I wrote this book and created the website www.drmichael.com so that more people may gain access to the medications they need at prices they can afford. Patients remind us daily of the money they have saved, as well as the improvement in the quality of their lives.

Although *Drugs for Less* contains a great deal of information, it is neither encyclopedic nor dogmatic. New drugs are approved each month, and both state and federal laws governing prescription drugs change frequently. Some physicians and pharmacists may disagree with some of its contents. The material in this book should form the basis of a discussion among you, your physician, and your pharmacist. Not all approaches to a problem apply to everyone, and taking the wrong approach can lead to greater problems. You should take medication only after your physician performs a careful history and physical examination, makes a diagnosis, and, most important, writes a prescription. Your doctor is aware of the particulars of your medical condition and needs to supervise and approve any changes in your medical care. Do not under any circumstances alter any of your medications without the approval of your physician.

Drugs for Less aims to provide you with the tools you need to reduce your prescription drug costs. Its goal is not to give medical advice; that is the duty of your physician. Its goal is not to promote political solutions; that is the job of our elected representatives. Pursuit of a healthy life is your responsibility, which is best carried out in partnership with your doctors and other health care professionals. My sincere hope is that *Drugs for Less* will help you and your loved ones obtain the medications you need at prices you can afford.

Introduction

SEVEN STRATEGIES
FOR LOWERING YOUR DRUG COSTS

PRESCRIPTION DRUGS are indispensable to the practice of modern medicine and have greatly improved our length and quality of life. Americans born in 1900 had a life expectancy of less than fifty years. Now current life expectancy has increased to nearly eighty years. Pharmaceutical advances have created much of that improvement. Diabetes and many infections were lethal before the discovery of insulin and penicillin. High blood pressure medications have greatly reduced the risk of developing heart attack and stroke. Potent antiulcer drugs have nearly eliminated the need for surgery to remove an ulcer-riddled stomach. Antidepressant and antipsychotic drugs have steadily advanced the treatment of depression and psychosis. Tylenol® and Advil® relieve headaches and muscle pains for millions of people. Hugh Hefner brags on national television about his active sex life thanks to the wonders of Viagra®.

Pharmaceutical drugs have transformed modern life, and consumers' demand for these products appears limitless. What wouldn't you pay for medications to improve your health or to lengthen your life by thirty years? You would probably pay whatever you could afford. The problem is that a growing number of people cannot afford the high cost of drugs today.

In my work as a cardiologist, I meet many patients who are suffering due to their inability to afford medications. Patients across the United States are repeatedly admitted into hospitals because they have stopped taking their drugs. Some patients even endure strokes or heart attacks. All of them understand the vital importance of taking medication to maintain their health. They know that life without health is a wretched bargain. Many live in fear that their life, or a loved one's life, will end prematurely because their medications are not affordable.

The elderly who live on fixed incomes are particularly affected by the rising costs. Some are even forced to choose between buying food and buying their medications. Senior citizens living in the northern United States frequently take bus trips to Canada to purchase drugs at discounted prices even though this practice violates current U.S. law. Those living in the South and the West travel to Mexico for the same purpose. Purchasing medications from other countries has gained such widespread support that Congress has considered changing the law governing drug importation.

The number of Americans without health insurance has reached 45 million. Millions of men and women working full-time lack health insurance and struggle to purchase the drugs they need. Due to the expense, some uninsured patients do not seek medical care until a medical catastrophe strikes.

But the poor and uninsured are not alone. The soaring cost of prescription drugs also affects those with excellent health insurance and prescription drug coverage. Those purchasing prescription drugs with private insurance are usually subjected to a tier system. Older generic drugs belong to a lower tier, are less expensive, and require lower monthly copayments. Newer and more expensive brand-name medications belong to a higher tier with correspondingly higher prices and higher monthly prescription drug copayments.

The tier system of paying for medications transfers some of the pharmaceutical cost from insurance companies to the individuals requiring the medications. A monthly copayment of $50 for each drug is charged for the higher-tiered medications. This $600 annual cost for one medication quickly grows into an annual cost exceeding $1,000 for patients requiring several medications.

Those who do not purchase medications still must pay higher insurance premiums each year, as insurers pass along their increasing costs of buying drugs. Companies paying for employees' health insurance must pass along these increased costs to employees by requiring higher deductibles and to their customers by raising prices. Major corporations are more likely to outsource jobs to workers in other countries in part to avoid paying for rising health care benefits. *Thus all Americans, rich and poor alike, are directly or indirectly affected by rising prescription drug costs.*

The federal government, state governments, and cities are all affected by rising drug costs. Medicaid and Medicare are large governmental health care programs enacted in the 1960s to pay for health care. State and federal governments jointly fund Medicaid, and the federal government funds Medicare. Medicaid provides health care to certain low-income Americans, and Medicare provides health care to elderly Americans. Eligibility for these programs has grown, and now tens of millions of Americans are entitled to Medicare or Medicaid.

Medicaid currently provides prescription drug coverage, and Medicare will begin offering prescription drug insurance in 2006. The Medicare Prescription Drug, Improvement and Modernization Act provides a voluntary prescription drug benefit for Medicare recipients. Although this Medicare drug benefit plan is the largest entitlement plan enacted in more than thirty years, it will pay for only a fraction of seniors' prescription drug cost. The plan shifts a portion of the payment for prescription drugs to taxpayers, but it does not slow the rising cost of drugs, nor does it assist the 240 million Americans who do not have Medicare benefits.

The legal obligation of state Medicaid programs to pay for recipients' prescription drugs has worsened many states' fiscal crisis. States purchase large quantities of medications for poor residents via the Medicaid program, and they also feel the effects of rising drug costs.

States have responded to this problem in a variety of ways. Maine passed a state law establishing a program called Maine Rx that lowers prescription drug prices for residents lacking prescription drug coverage. Maine Rx requires drug manufacturers to sell medications to Maine residents who lack prescription drug insurance at the same deeply discounted price at which they sell drugs to Maine's Medicaid recipients. The Pharmaceutical Research and Manufacturers of America (PhRMA), the pharmaceutical manufacturers' trade group, sued Maine, stating that Maine Rx would illegally interfere with interstate commerce. Ultimately, the Supreme Court ruled in favor of Maine. Other states are expected to develop similar programs.

Some states are moving ahead with programs to help residents import cheaper drugs from Canada by placing links on their websites to assist residents in purchasing drugs. These states include Minnesota (www.state.mn.us/cgi-bin/portal/mn/jsp/home.do?agency=Rx) and Wisconsin (www.drugsavings.wi.gov). Illinois's governor, Rod Blagojevich, recently announced a plan named I-SaveRx to provide access to prescription drugs from several countries. Its website, www.i-saverx.net, is open to all Illinois, Wisconsin, Kansas, and Missouri residents to assist in the purchase of discounted pharmaceuticals from Canada, Ireland, and the United Kingdom. To learn more about I-SaveRx, go to the website or telephone 866-472-8333. Vermont has filed suit against the Food and Drug Administration to allow drug importation from Canada.

Cities are joining states in creating these programs. Springfield, Massachusetts', local government saved more than $2 million in its first year of offering its city employees the opportunity to purchase certain prescription medications from Canada. Its neighbor Boston is planning a similar program.

While the Medicare Prescription Drug, Improvement and Modernization Act will help some seniors better afford medications and state and local programs will help some residents, these measures probably won't help your problem of runaway drug prices now.

You can lower your drug costs today by becoming an informed consumer. The following chapters will give you the information you need to obtain your drugs at affordable prices. Adam Smith wrote about the "invisible hand" of capitalism; however, even the most dexterous hand needs direction from an educated mind. Consumers understand the relative value of one product compared to a similar product and spend their money accordingly. Capitalism thrives in an environment filled with transparent pricing and widespread consumer information. As airlines and computer manufacturers will attest, when these conditions exist, prices fall dramatically. The major reason that airline travel, computers, and many other consumer products are so competitively priced is that information about the products and their prices is widely available to consumers.

Additional information about the relative effectiveness and value of different medications is badly needed by consumers. Pharmacists generally provide materials discussing the prescribed drug at the time of purchase, but the information is limited mostly to indications for usage, side effects, contraindications with other medications, and directions for taking the pills. The overwhelming majority of consumers are largely uniformed about which other drugs might be alternatives. They do not have access to pharmaceutical price lists or studies comparing the relative effectiveness of various drugs.

By contrast, newspapers and magazines are filled with information about the best values in computers and airline travel. Articles list the products' relative merits as well as their prices. This widely disseminated information then enables consumers to purchase products more efficiently. Savvy travelers can now search multiple Internet websites for the best travel deals. Some travelers might fly to a different airport, take a later flight, or use connecting flights to their advantage. In other words, knowing how the system works empowers travelers, gives them multiple options, and makes traveling more affordable and accessible. This guidebook will show you how the drug delivery system works, which drugs can be sliced into two parts, which drugs have low-cost generic alternatives, and which pharmacies have the best prices. It will give you many ideas for other ways to save money.

Consider an example where informed consumers could save a lot of money. The National Institutes of Health studied thousands of patients with elevated blood pressure at an expense to taxpayers of tens of millions of dollars. The Antihypertensive and Lipid-Lowering Treatment to Prevent Heart Attack Trial (also known as the ALLHAT study), compared several popular medications used to treat high blood pressure. The trial determined that a generic medication, chlorthalidone, was equivalent (and in some ways superior) to the world's best-selling high blood pressure medication, Norvasc®. The daily cost of a dose of Norvasc® is about ten times greater than that of chlorthalidone.

Armed with information from the ALLHAT study, available at www.nhlbi.nih.gov/health/allhat/, consumers with elevated blood pressure could ask their physicians whether chlorthalidone is appropriate for them. Changing from one medication to the other could result in hundreds of dollars of savings every year.

The most proactive patients save the most money. If large numbers of consumers collectively become informed, dramatic savings will occur. After consumers in the northern United States discovered that pharmaceuticals were priced less expensively in Canada, this information was initially shared among seniors, then ultimately disseminated widely by the media. Consumers have collectively reduced their annual pharmaceutical costs by hundreds of millions of dollars by purchasing medications from Canadian pharmacies. Sir Francis Bacon's declaration that "knowledge is power" seems more relevant today than ever before. The information contained in *Drugs for Less* has saved my patients hundreds of thousands of dollars. But, more important for many, the peace of mind of knowing that they will get the medications they need is the greatest benefit. *Drugs for Less* offers seven practical steps to help you lower your drug bills. The first step of this journey begins with an overview of those seven strategies.

Strategy 1: Learn Prices

You certainly know how much you pay the pharmacy to buy your medications, but you do not know if you are getting a good deal. This chapter shows you how U.S. consumers pay vastly *different* prices for the *same* drug. It also gives you prices for different dosages of best-selling drugs, so you can begin to know if you are paying a full, retail price when you could be paying less.

Strategy 2: Comparison Shop

Although you comparison shop for the best price on travel, computers, groceries, and gasoline, you likely buy your drugs from the most convenient pharmacy. After learning how to comparison shop for your prescription drugs, you will be able to dramatically lower your monthly cost of those drugs. This chapter will teach you how to save money by buying larger quantities of drugs, using the Internet to compare prices, and—if you decide to buy your medications from Canada—ways of doing this as safely as possible.

Strategy 3: Buy Generic Medications

The major difference between generic medications and brand-name medications is price. Generic medications are safe and regulated by the FDA to the same specifications as brand-name medications, but generics can cost 90 percent less than their brand-name equivalents. They are one of the highest-value, lowest-cost bargains available in prescription drugs. This chapter gives possible generic substitutions for brand-name drugs for common ailments as well as the names of more than 150 useful generic medications. Many readers will qualify for a program to purchase over fifty generic medications at a cost of about $1.00 a week.

Strategy 4: Slice Medications

Years ago, male patients began to ask me to write their Viagra prescription for the 100 mg tablets, even though all they needed was a 50 mg dose. They had realized that the 100 mg tablets were priced identically to the 50 mg tablets, and therefore they would buy the 100 mg tablets and slice them into two parts. For many men, both the 50 mg and 100 mg tablets treated their erectile dysfunction equally well, so my patients would effectively "buy one, get one free." While this strategy will not work for all medications, it will work for many of the world's best-selling drugs; a list of one hundred drugs suitable for slicing is presented.

Strategy 5: Consider Other Medications in the Same Class

Smart shoppers know what they are buying, and informed patients understand how their medications work. Medications are grouped into classes in terms of how they work. By knowing about different classes of drugs, you will learn if there are lower-cost alternatives available. Major classes of drugs are listed, as well as which drugs within a class have a generic substitute available and which are available without a prescription.

Strategy 6: Put Your Government to Work for You

Federal and state governments are the number one purchasers of health care and prescription drugs, and you may qualify for assistance in paying for your prescription drugs. Many veterans do not realize that they can receive prescription drugs for free or at deeply discounted prices. People who are entitled to Medicaid are also entitled to the program's prescription drug benefits, and this chapter shows you how to determine if you qualify for your state's program. The new Medicare drug program, and how it will affect your wallet, is discussed. Phone numbers and websites for many state assistance programs are also listed.

Strategy 7: Use Pharmaceutical Assistance Programs

Hundreds of my patients have benefited by being enrolled in the pharmaceutical companies' assistance programs. These programs provide free or extremely discounted medications for patients meeting program requirements. A listing of hundreds of such medications is provided, as well as details about the individual programs.

PART I

THE SEVEN STRATEGIES

STRATEGY 1

LEARN PRICES

A MERICANS ARE THE WORLD'S GREATEST comparison shoppers. We know the price of virtually every product. Our longest-running, highest-rated daytime television game show is *The Price Is Right*, now in its thirty-second year. Despite our collective expertise with value shopping, however, few consumers know if they're getting their medications at the best possible price.

Unlike virtually all other consumer products, prescription drugs have opaque pricing, that is consumers do not have ready access to information about their prices. For example, airline travel was opaquely priced thirty years ago; consequently, in the 1970s flights were expensive, poorly advertised, and not readily available. Today airline travel is transparently priced, with individual flight prices widely available on the Internet, and the cost of airline travel has plummeted.

Because there is no widely available pharmaceutical price guide available in book form or on the Internet and because drug prices are not widely advertised, it is difficult to know how much medications cost. Furthermore, very few consumers understand the complex drug distribution system. This chapter will help you understand pharmaceutical pricing and provide you with the prices of many drugs.

How Drugs Are Priced

Drug pricing is much more straightforward in many other countries in the world, particularly Canada, where the prices of pharmaceuticals are regulated. Canada's Patented Medicine Prices Review Board (PMPRB) establishes the maximum price charged for a prescription medication. In general terms, the PMPRB mandates that the price

— 3 —

charged for almost any new drug does not exceed the price of the most expensive drug treating that disease. The PMPRB thus helps ensure that pharmaceutical prices in Canada are not the highest in the world. Readers interested in how the Canadian government reduces the prices of brand-name drugs can learn more from the PMPRB website, www.pmprb-cepmb.gc.ca.

The price paid for brand-name prescription drugs in the United States varies widely due to a complex distribution system involving many middlemen. An April 2000 study by the Department of Health and Human Services, "Report to the President: Prescription Drug Coverage, Spending, Utilization and Prices," explains how pharmaceuticals travel from the manufacturing plant, to retail pharmacies, and then to consumers, and who pays how much for what along the way. The report may be found in its entirety at aspe.hhs.gov/health/reports/drugstudy/. Public awareness about brand-name prescription drug pricing could have the same effect that public awareness about airline travel pricing had years ago. How can anyone choose low-cost, high-quality medications without first knowing the prices of the drugs?

Pharmaceutical manufacturers, such as Pfizer and Merck, produce drugs that contain active ingredients. The actual cost of producing an active ingredient is small; most of the cost goes into research, development, and promotion of the drug. The April 2002 issue of *Life Extension* magazine stated that brand-name medications are priced 40 to 300 times as much as the cost of their ingredients. The additional cost funds the safety studies required to meet FDA requirements, as well as for marketing, research, and other costs borne by the pharmaceutical companies, and earns the companies a profit.

Manufacturers then ship the majority of their products to wholesalers, which purchase large quantities and resell them to tens of thousands of retail pharmacies across the United States. The price paid to the manufacturer for the pharmaceuticals is called the *manufacturer's price*. Manufacturers also sell pharmaceuticals at substantially reduced prices to a few other large buyers, such as the federal government for veterans' hospitals and large teaching hospitals. Although the federal government obtains the best prices for drugs sold in the United States, the Medicare Prescription Drug, Improvement and Modernization Act prohibits the federal government from negotiating discounts for Medicare beneficiaries.

Retail pharmacies purchase pharmaceuticals from wholesalers at the *acquisition price*. These include independent pharmacies, mail-order pharmacies, chain pharmacies, as well as pharmacies located in groceries and mass merchandisers. The pharmacy adds its costs, including rent, utilities, salaries, prescription-filling costs, and profit. It then sells the drug to consumers at the *retail pharmacy price*. Consumers then purchase pharmaceuticals from a pharmacy in one of four ways.

Four Ways of Buying Prescription Drugs and Who Pays

Four patients illustrate how much is paid for a typical brand-name medication. Alice is a 42-year-old uninsured, homeless woman with an extremely weak heart. She lives in a shelter and has not received any benefits such as Medicare or Medicaid. She is one of the growing numbers of uninsured, and this group has tens of millions of members. Brad is a 62-year-old Vietnam veteran who was insured during combat and receives full disability coverage. His medications, as well as his entire medical care, are provided by the local veterans' hospital. Carol is a 34-year-old mother covered by Medicaid. This state and federal government program pays for most of her health care and prescription drugs. Dan is the retired 58-year-old CFO of a Fortune 500 company that pays for his health care and prescriptions through private health insurance. By coincidence, all of them need to take the same brand-name drug, Stayfit. Alice, Carol, and Dan purchase it at the pharmacy near my office. Brad obtains his at the nearby veterans' hospital pharmacy. (The patients' names, as well as the drug Stayfit, are fictional.)

Stayfit comes in only one dosage and is taken once daily. A monthly supply of Stayfit has an average wholesale price, better known as the AWP, of $50. The AWP is terribly named, as no one actually seems to pay the AWP. Wholesalers purchase pharmaceuticals from manufacturers at the *manufacturer's price* and then sell to pharmacies at the *acquisition price*. Retail pharmacies then sell the medications to their customers at the *retail pharmacy price*. For informed consumers, the AWP of a drug is somewhat analogous to the full sticker price of a car—an inflated price that uninformed buyers pay. For informed shoppers, it is merely a starting price from which to seek discounts. The Red Book®

lists the AWP for all pharmaceuticals and is published annually by the Thomson Corporation. This comprehensive price guide, usually used by pharmacists, may be purchased for about $70 by telephoning 800-678-5689.

CASH CUSTOMERS

The first of our four groups of consumers comprises those customers who pay in full at the time of the transaction; they are called *cash customers*. Alice, our 42-year-old uninsured patient, is in this group. Cash customers make up about one-third of all pharmaceutical consumers. Tens of millions of Americans are in this group, including many Medicare beneficiaries, people without health insurance, and those with health insurance but without pharmaceutical benefits. Medicare does not currently pay for prescription drugs but will do so beginning in 2006. The Medicare prescription drug plan is discussed in more detail in Strategy 6, "Put Your Government to Work for You."

Alice gets her supply of Stayfit at her local pharmacy. Generally, wholesalers pay 20 percent less than the AWP, so the pharmaceutical company receives $40 from the wholesaler (AWP minus 20 percent). The wholesaler adds a 2 to 4 percent markup—in this example, $1 (or a 2.5 percent markup)—then sells it to the retail pharmacy for $41. This is the acquisition price. The pharmacy charges its cash customers the AWP plus a markup, generally 4 percent. So Alice pays $52, the full retail price, to her local pharmacy, and experiences sticker shock at how expensive the drug is.

VETERANS

Brad, the 62-year-old disabled veteran, pays the pharmacy nothing for his medications. The medication is dispensed directly by the veterans' hospital or a pharmacy located on a military base; no wholesalers or retail pharmacies are involved. Acting on behalf of the federal government, veterans' hospitals negotiate large discounts from drug companies. These vary from drug to drug; for Stayfit, the discount is 52 percent, which is typical. So the government pays the manufacturer $24 on Brad's behalf (AWP minus 52 percent).

The Veterans Health Care Act of 1992 mandated that any pharmaceuticals purchased by the Medicaid program must also be made available for purchase by veterans hospitals at prices set by the Federal

Supply Schedule, also known as the FSS prices. The FSS price of any drug must be equal to or lower than the best price offered by the drug company to any other buyers under similar conditions. These prices are available online in database format at www.vapbm.org/PBM/ prices.htm. Veterans' hospitals, the Department of Defense, the Coast Guard, the U.S. Public Health Service, Indian tribes, and a few other organizations may purchase pharmaceuticals at these prices. Purchases by these entities account for about 2 percent of the sales of all prescription drugs.

MEDICAID BENEFICIARIES

Carol, the 34-year-old mother with Medicaid benefits, also pays nothing when she fills her prescription at the pharmacy. Other Medicaid recipients might have a nominal copayment ranging from 50 cents to $2, depending upon their individual state's program.

Medicaid pricing is more complicated than the first two types of pricing. The Omnibus Budget Reconciliation Act of 1990 requires pharmaceutical manufacturers to rebate money to Medicaid for any pharmaceuticals purchased by Medicaid beneficiaries through retail pharmacies. These rebates vary but average approximately 20 percent of the manufacturer's price. This method of reimbursement allows those with Medicaid benefits to access the large retail pharmacy network, while providing a price discount to the Medicaid program, which is funded by state and federal tax dollars.

In Carol's case, the manufacturer sells Stayfit to the wholesaler for $40; the wholesaler sells it to the pharmacy for $41. Medicaid then pays the pharmacy its acquisition cost, plus a dispensing fee of about $4.50, for a total of $45.50. The pharmaceutical manufacturer then rebates 20 percent of the manufacturer's price to Medicaid. In this case, the rebate would be $8 (20 percent of the $40 that the manufacturer originally was paid).

After all the transactions are completed, the net payments are as follows: Carol pays nothing. The wholesaler receives $1. The manufacturer receives a net of $32 (the $40 manufacturer's price less the 20 percent rebate). The Medicaid program pays a net of $37.50 ($45.50 initial pharmacy payment minus the $8 manufacturer rebate, which is subsequently reimbursed). The pharmacy receives a net payment of $4.50, its dispensing fee.

Whew! I told you that understanding Medicaid pricing was tough—but private health insurance drug pricing is even more convoluted and complex.

PERSONS WITH PRIVATE HEALTH INSURANCE

Dan, the retired 58-year-old CFO patient, pays a $20 copayment when he purchases Stayfit from his local pharmacy. Despite his extensive expertise in finance, Dan has no information about the payment system for those with private health insurance and prescription drug coverage. More than 60 percent of Americans receive employer-based coverage, making this the largest group of consumers. Their health insurer also pays a portion of the pharmaceutical cost; however, the amount that the insurer pays is less than Dan realizes, due to the convoluted payment procedure. The vast majority of health insurers provide their enrollees with pharmaceutical benefits through large companies known as pharmacy benefit managers (PBMs).

PBMs provide many services for health plans, including negotiating price discounts with pharmacies and negotiating discounts and rebates with drug manufacturers. They also operate mail-order pharmacies and manage claims data, thus allowing insurers to provide their members with the ability to buy prescription drugs at a discounted rate.

PBMs exert tremendous control over prescription practices by developing drug formularies, running mail-order fulfillment centers, and contracting with retail pharmacies. Drug formularies are large lists of drugs put together by insurers and PBMs. Generic drugs are most preferred and priced in a lower tier (i.e., at a cheaper price), while brand-name drugs are in a higher tier. Sometimes, if a drug is not on formulary, the insurer will not pay for it. Fortunately, Stayfit is on formulary as a middle-tier drug so Dan's copayment is not the $50 required for the higher-tier drugs.

The three largest PBMs—Caremark, Express Scripts, and Medco Health Solutions—account for more than 80 percent of the PBM market. Collectively, these companies greatly influence which drugs the tens of millions of Americans with prescription drug insurance take. Many lawsuits have been filed that accuse the PBMs of multiple legal and ethical violations. In April 2004, Medco Health Solutions, the largest PBM, settled a case with twenty states in which it had been accused of pressuring doctors to switch medications. In settling, Medco denied any violation of unfair trade practices.

Drug manufacturers pay PBMs cash rebates for placing their pharmaceuticals into the formularies of various health plans. Also, it is claimed that PBMs generally pay retail pharmacies about 2 percent less than PBMs charge health plans for the pharmaceuticals, thus creating another profit source. Since PBMs do not disclose the financial specifics of their relationship with manufacturers or pharmacies, the actual prices provided in the following example are only illustrative.

Returning to the example of our retired CFO patient, Dan, the prices paid are as follows: The pharmaceutical company receives $40 from the wholesaler (AWP minus 20 percent) but rebates money to the PBM. The rebate paid by the manufacturer to the PBM varies from 5 percent to 35 percent; however, assuming a rebate of 20 percent of the manufacturer's price, the manufacturer nets $32 ($40 minus $8 rebate). The wholesaler again makes $1 by purchasing the pharmaceutical from the manufacturer for $40 and selling it to the retail pharmacy for $41.

The net price paid to the retail pharmacy is dictated primarily by the pharmacy's contract with the PBM. On average, the pharmacy receives a total of $46 (AWP minus 13 percent plus a $2.50 dispensing fee) and makes a profit of $5. The PBM pays the pharmacy its contracted price less the amount the customer paid as a copayment. In this case the copayment was $20. The PBM receives money from the insurer for its services as well as money from the manufacturer in the form of a rebate. The PBM reportedly passes on 70 to 90 percent of the manufacturer's rebate to the insurer. The net amount paid by the PBM is $18 ($46 pharmacy cost less $20 customer copayment minus the $8 manufacturer rebate)—$2 less than the consumer's $20 copayment.

The pharmacy's sales ticket may list Stayfit's original sales price at $52, the price paid by cash customers. Having paid only a $20 copayment for a $52 medication, Dan thought that his prescription drug coverage was a great deal. But in fact he pays more than one-half of the actual cost of the drug with his copayment. Dan, a financially erudite patient, was not happy to learn that he was not getting such a great deal.

Summing Up

The following table summarizes the cost of purchasing Stayfit with its AWP of $50. The prices are illustrative, not exact.

Prices Paid for a $50 Brand-Name Drug Based on Insurance				
	NO DRUG INSURANCE	PRIVATE INSURANCE	MEDICAID BENEFITS	VETERANS BENEFITS
List price (AWP)	$50.00	$50.00	$50.00	$50.00
Manufacturer's price (how much the drug company was initially paid)	$40.00	$40.00	$40.00	$24.00
Acquisition price (how much the wholesaler paid)	$41.00	$41.00	$41.00	Not Applicable
Retail price (the total price paid to the pharmacy)	$52.00	$46.00	$45.50	Not Applicable
Pharmacy profit	$11.00	$5.00	$4.50	Not Applicable
Manufacturer's profit (how much the company was paid after rebates and discounts)	$40.00	$32.00	$32.00	$24.00
Amount paid by consumer at time of purchase	$52.00	$20.00 copayment	Nominal copayment	$0.00
Amount paid by third party	$0.00	$18.00	$37.50	$24.00
Total amount paid for drug	$52.00	$38.00	$37.50	$24.00

Source: Adapted from "Report to the President. Prescription Drug Coverage, Spending, Utilization, and Prices." From the department of Health & Human Services, April 2000 and available at http://aspe.hhs.gov/health/reports/drugstudy/.

The table illustrates four major points about the complex arrangements of purchasing pharmaceuticals. First, different consumers pay widely varying amounts of money for identical medications depending on whether they have Medicare, Medicaid, veterans' benefits, or private health insurance with drug coverage. The complexity helps to keep drug prices a secret, since different people pay different prices for the same drug, and those with insurance do not know the total amount that is paid for their drugs.

Second, those without health insurance and those with Medicare pay the most. Cash customers pay 25 percent more to the drug manufacturers and provide double the profit for the pharmacy compared to those with health insurance. A report published in June 2004 by Families USA, *One in Three: Non-Elderly Americans Without Health Insurance, 2002–2003*, stated that "approximately 81.8 million people—one out of three (32.2 percent) of those under the age of 65—were without health insurance for all or part of 2002 and 2003."

Third, patients with private health insurance and prescription drug coverage pay a much larger percentage of the total pharmaceutical price paid than they realize. In Dan's case, he paid for more than 50 percent of the total cost at the point of service. If his copayment had been higher or the rebate from the manufacturer to the PBM had been larger, he would have paid for nearly all of the cost of the medication. By increasing Dan's copayment, the insurer shifts the drug costs to Dan and increases its profit.

Fourth, those with Medicaid or veterans' health benefits pay little or nothing at the point of service for their medications. However, the government pays very different prices depending on whether the medications are for Medicaid beneficiaries or veterans. As taxpaying citizens, we should want the government to pay the lowest prices available for *all* beneficiaries since all of the drugs are paid for with tax dollars.

Currently, the federal government pays the lowest amount when medications are purchased by the Veterans Health Administration. In the example on the previous page, which excludes the cost of running a pharmacy, the price paid by the Veterans Health Administration for pharmaceuticals was about 36 percent less than the total cost paid by Medicaid: ($37.50-$24)/$37.50.

As of 2006, Medicare recipients will be eligible to purchase prescription drug insurance, and the federal government will be spending additional billions of dollars on prescription drugs. The new Medicare law states that private companies will administer this pharmaceutical benefit and that the government cannot negotiate price discounts from manufacturers. Unless this provision of the law is changed, it is very likely that the taxpayers' cost of purchasing medications will be higher for Medicare recipients than for those with Medicaid or veterans' health benefits.

Average Wholesale Prices

The following table gives the acquisition price and the average wholesale price (AWP) of many commonly prescribed brand-name medications. This list was obtained from a metropolitan Atlanta pharmacy pricing list in late 2004, so the prices are not exactly the same as those published in the *Red Book*®. The price you pay at the pharmacy—the pharmacy's retail price—will likely be higher than the pharmacy's acquisition price but may be lower than the AWP. As Strategy 2, "Comparison Shop," details, prices vary widely among pharmacies; nonetheless, this table provides you with a general idea of the cost for a single dose of many of the best-selling brand-name drugs as well as the AWP.

Note that many of the drugs have the same price for different dosages. In Strategy 4, "Slice Medications," you'll learn how to use this information to calculate your cost per dosage and perhaps save money by changing your dose or slicing your medication.

Prices of Commonly Prescribed Brand-Name Pharmaceuticals

BRAND NAME	STRENGTH	NUMBER OF TABLETS	ACQUISITION PRICE	ACQUISITION PRICE PER TABLET	AVERAGE WHOLESALE PRICE (AWP)	AWP PER TABLET
Accupril®	10 mg	90	$97.85	$1.09	$122.31	$1.36
Accupril®	20 mg	90	$97.85	$1.09	$122.31	$1.36
Accupril®	40 mg	90	$97.85	$1.09	$122.31	$1.36
Aciphex®	20 mg	30	$112.58	$3.75	$135.10	$4.50
Actos®	15 mg	90	$271.23	$3.01	$330.90	$3.68
Actos®	30 mg	90	$434.28	$4.83	$529.82	$5.89
Actos®	45 mg	30	$157.02	$5.23	$191.56	$6.39
Altace®	5 mg	100	$123.60	$1.24	$150.79	$1.51
Altace®	10 mg	100	$151.69	$1.52	$185.06	$1.85
Amaryl®	2 mg	100	$54.67	$0.55	$68.34	$0.68
Amaryl®	4 mg	100	$103.11	$1.03	$128.89	$1.29
Aricept®	5 mg	90	$373.41	$4.15	$455.56	$5.06
Aricept®	10 mg	90	$373.41	$4.15	$455.56	$5.06
Atacand®	8 mg	30	$40.79	$1.36	$49.76	$1.66
Atacand®	16 mg	100	$136.04	$1.36	$165.97	$1.66
Atacand®	32 mg	100	$184.01	$1.84	$224.49	$2.24
Avandia®	4 mg	100	$251.34	$2.51	$314.18	$3.14
Avandia®	8 mg	100	$465.49	$4.65	$581.86	$5.82
Avapro®	150 mg	100	$137.05	$1.37	$167.20	$1.67
Avapro®	300 mg	30	$49.43	$1.65	$60.30	$2.01
Bextra®	10 mg	100	$263.81	$2.64	$329.76	$3.30
Bextra®	20 mg	100	$263.81	$2.64	$329.76	$3.30

Prices of Commonly Prescribed Brand-Name Pharmaceuticals cont.

BRAND NAME	STRENGTH	NUMBER OF TABLETS	ACQUISITION PRICE	ACQUISITION PRICE PER TABLET	AVERAGE WHOLESALE PRICE (AWP)	AWP PER TABLET
Celebrex®	100 mg	100	$151.89	$1.52	$189.86	$1.90
Celebrex®	200 mg	100	$249.13	$2.49	$311.41	$3.11
Celexa®	20 mg	100	$227.79	$2.28	$277.90	$2.78
Celexa®	40 mg	100	$237.71	$2.38	$290.01	$2.90
Coreg®	3.125 mg	100	$152.76	$1.53	$190.95	$1.91
Coreg®	6.25 mg	100	$152.76	$1.53	$190.95	$1.91
Coreg®	12.5 mg	100	$152.76	$1.53	$190.95	$1.91
Coreg®	25 mg	100	$152.76	$1.53	$190.95	$1.91
Cozaar®	50 mg	100	$138.91	$1.39	$169.47	$1.69
Cozaar®	100 mg	100	$189.22	$1.89	$230.85	$2.31
Diovan®	80 mg	100	$143.14	$1.43	$174.63	$1.75
Diovan®	160 mg	100	$153.90	$1.54	$187.76	$1.88
Diovan®	320 mg	100	$194.70	$1.95	$237.53	$2.38
Effexor XR®	37.5 mg	100	$243.30	$2.43	$304.13	$3.04
Effexor XR®	75 mg	100	$272.55	$2.73	$340.69	$3.41
Effexor XR®	150 mg	100	$296.85	$2.97	$371.06	$3.71
Evista®	60 mg	100	$241.15	$2.41	$289.38	$2.89
Fosamax®	70 mg	4	$61.52	$15.38	$75.05	$18.76
Lipitor®	10 mg	100	$217.05	$2.17	$271.31	$2.71
Lipitor®	20 mg	100	$314.94	$3.15	$393.68	$3.94
Lipitor®	40 mg	90	$269.95	$3.00	$337.44	$3.75

Prices of Commonly Prescribed Brand-Name Pharmaceuticals cont.

BRAND NAME	STRENGTH	NUMBER OF TABLETS	ACQUISITION PRICE	ACQUISITION PRICE PER TABLET	AVERAGE WHOLESALE PRICE (AWP)	AWP PER TABLET
Lipitor®	80 mg	90	$269.95	$3.00	$337.44	$3.75
Lotensin®	10 mg	100	$93.43	$0.93	$113.98	$1.14
Lotensin®	20 mg	100	$93.43	$0.93	$113.98	$1.14
Lotensin®	40 mg	100	$93.43	$0.93	$113.98	$1.14
Mavik®	1 mg	100	$95.84	$0.96	$119.80	$1.20
Mavik®	2 mg	100	$95.84	$0.96	$119.80	$1.20
Mavik®	4 mg	100	$95.84	$0.96	$119.80	$1.20
Micardis®	40 mg	30	$41.34	$1.38	$50.43	$1.68
Micardis®	80 mg	30	$44.34	$1.48	$54.09	$1.80
Neurontin®	100 mg	100	$47.33	$0.47	$59.16	$0.59
Neurontin®	300 mg	100	$118.32	$1.18	$147.90	$1.48
Nexium®	20 mg	100	$395.67	$3.96	$482.72	$4.83
Nexium®	40 mg	100	$395.67	$3.96	$482.72	$4.83
Norvasc®	5 mg	100	$132.15	$1.32	$165.19	$1.65
Norvasc®	10 mg	100	$181.35	$1.81	$226.69	$2.27
Paxil®	10 mg	30	$73.41	$2.45	$91.76	$3.06
Paxil®	20 mg	100	$260.58	$2.61	$325.73	$3.26
Paxil®	30 mg	30	$78.91	$2.63	$98.64	$3.29
Plavix®	75 mg	100	$363.97	$3.64	$444.04	$4.44
Remeron®	15 mg	30	$79.08	$2.64	$96.48	$3.22
Reminyl®	4 mg	60	$137.17	$2.29	$164.60	$2.74

Prices of Commonly Prescribed Brand-Name Pharmaceuticals cont.

BRAND NAME	STRENGTH	NUMBER OF TABLETS	ACQUISITION PRICE	ACQUISITION PRICE PER TABLET	AVERAGE WHOLESALE PRICE (AWP)	AWP PER TABLET
Reminyl®	8 mg	60	$137.17	$2.29	$164.60	$2.74
Reminyl®	12 mg	60	$137.17	$2.29	$164.60	$2.74
Viagra®	50 mg	100	$850.60	$8.51	$1,063.25	$10.63
Viagra®	100 mg	100	$850.60	$8.51	$1,063.25	$10.63
Zocor®	20 mg	100	$382.95	$3.83	$467.20	$4.67
Zocor®	40 mg	100	$382.95	$3.83	$467.20	$4.67
Zocor®	80 mg	100	$382.95	$3.83	$467.20	$4.67
Zoloft®	50 mg	100	$229.88	$2.30	$287.35	$2.87
Zoloft®	100 mg	100	$229.88	$2.30	$287.35	$2.87
Zyrtec®	10 mg	100	$175.94	$1.76	$219.93	$2.20

STRATEGY 2

COMPARISON SHOP

SAVVY CONSUMERS shop for bargains on computers, automobiles, gasoline, and almost every consumer product except medications. This chapter tells you how to save money on drugs by comparison shopping, and shows you the value of purchasing some medications in bulk quantity. The benefits and risks of purchasing pharmaceuticals online, including information about Canadian pharmacies, are discussed. Start saving money today by smart shopping for drugs.

Comparison Shopping at Various Types of Pharmacies, Between Different Quantities of Drugs, and Between Generic and Brand-Name Drugs

Chain pharmacies, independent pharmacies, grocery stores, and large discount retailers all sell drugs. As with other consumer goods, the same drugs sell for different prices at different stores. For instance, discount retailers such as Costco often sell medications at lower prices. Some groceries give an additional discount one day a week to seniors. If you purchase your medications at the local, most convenient pharmacy, you may not be saving as much as you could by shopping around. Internet websites such as Destination Rx™, www.destinationrx.com, compare prices among different online pharmacies and provide a range of prices for varying amounts of different drug dosages for U.S. online pharmacies. Some searches return a small number of online pharmacies to choose from, so be sure to check prices at www.costco.com, www.drugstore.com, and www.familymeds.com. Prices from these websites are presented throughout the book.

An uncommon place to check prices for your prescription drugs is with the Pequot Indian tribe in Connecticut. Native American Indians can buy prescription drugs from them at deeply discounted prices by using their website www.prxn.com or telephoning the pharmacy at 800-342-5779. Those who are not native American Indians must belong to a group such as AAA to use the pharmacy, and the drug prices are not as deeply discounted. I told a patient who is an Indian chief about this pharmacy, and he reported that the service was helpful for members of his tribe.

Once you've found the store with the best prices, compare prices among different quantities of drugs to see how much you will save by buying in bulk. Also, you can save an amazing amount by buying generic drugs, a topic we will touch on in this chapter and cover in much more depth in Strategy 3. Let's see how super savers shop.

In November 2004, Ed, an extraordinary shopper, compared prices at a local chain pharmacy and a local discount retailer for three drugs that belong in everyone's medicine chest: Advil®, aspirin, and Zantac®. These drugs are available for sale virtually everywhere. The generic name of Advil® is ibuprofen and the generic name of Zantac® is ranitidine. He started by comparing the prices of brand-name Advil® and generic ibuprofen, in small and large quantities.

Prices of Different Quantities of Brand-Name Advil® Versus Generic Ibuprofen at a Large Chain Drugstore

BRAND NAME: ADVIL®, 200MG			GENERIC: IBUPROFEN, 200 MG		
NUMBER OF TABLETS	PRICE	PRICE PER TABLET	NUMBER OF TABLETS	PRICE	PRICE PER TABLET
24	$4.19	$0.17	24	$2.99	$0.12
50	$5.99	$0.12	50	$4.99	$0.10
100	$8.99	$0.09	100	$7.39	$0.07

The above comparison demonstrates the high price paid for a small amount of a brand-name drug. The cost of a single brand-name

Advil® 200 mg tablet was 17 cents when purchased in a bottle of 24 but just 9 cents when purchased in a bottle of 100 tablets. Buying the generic ibuprofen instead of brand-name Advil® further increased your savings. Most remarkably, at Costco pharmacy the cost of 750 generic ibuprofen 200 mg tablets was just $6.79—less than one penny for each 200 mg tablet.

Prices of Different Quantities of Bayer Aspirin Versus Generic Aspirin at a Large Chain Drugstore					
BRAND NAME: BAYER ASPIRIN, 325 MG			GENERIC: ASPIRIN, 325 MG		
NUMBER OF TABLETS	PRICE	PRICE PER TABLET	NUMBER OF TABLETS	PRICE	PRICE PER TABLET
50	$5.19	$0.10	120	$2.69	$0.02
200	$9.79	$0.05	300	$4.49	$0.01

Sales of brand-name Bayer aspirin continue despite the widespread availability of the less expensive generic aspirin. The difference in cost between brand-name Bayer aspirin and generic aspirin is substantial. When purchased in a bottle of 200 tablets, a single 325 mg Bayer aspirin costs almost 5 cents, whereas a single generic aspirin in a bottle of 300 tablets costs less than 2 cents. Costco pharmacy charges $3.59 for a 1,000-tablet bottle of generic 325 mg aspirin; this is less than a penny for each 325 mg tablet.

Prices of Different Quantities of Brand-Name Zantac® Versus Generic Ranitidine at a Large Chain Drugstore					
BRAND NAME: ZANTAC®, 75 MG			GENERIC: RANITIDINE, 75 MG		
NUMBER OF TABLETS	PRICE	PRICE PER TABLET	NUMBER OF TABLETS	PRICE	PRICE PER TABLET
20	$8.79	$0.44	20	$6.69	$0.33
60	$14.99	$0.25	60	$14.19	$0.24
80	$21.99	$0.27	80	$17.99	$0.22

The total amount of money saved is more for Zantac®. A 75 mg tablet of Zantac® costs about 44 cents per tablet when purchased in a bottle of 20 tablets and about 27 cents per tablet when purchased in a bottle of 80 tablets. Generic ranitidine costs about 22 cents per tablet when purchased in a bottle of 80 tablets. Costco pharmacy charges $5.99 for a 240-tablet bottle of generic ranitidine 75 mg tablets; this is less than three cents for each 75 mg tablet.

These three examples make three major points about shopping for pharmaceuticals. First, it is cheaper to buy in volume quantities. Instead of focusing as much on the price for a bottle of medications, focus more on the price-per-tablet. Second, it is cheaper to buy generic rather than brand-name drugs. This is discussed further in Strategy 3. Third, different stores mark up prices by widely different amounts and it is generally cheaper to buy from a discount retailer. You should check prices at stand-alone pharmacies such as Eckerd, CVS, and Walgreens, pharmacies in superstores such as Costco and SAM'S Club, and online pharmacies to find the lowest price. The examples were of over-the-counter drugs; however, comparison shopping should be done for prescription drugs as well.

Although Costco requires a club membership (which costs $45 annually) to purchase other merchandise, membership is not required to buy pharmaceuticals inside its warehouses using cash or a debit card. You must have a Costco membership to purchase pharmaceuticals through the Internet. For those with very high prescription drug bills, the Costco Executive Membership may further decrease costs. This type of membership, which costs $100 per year, provides a 2 percent rebate on all Costco purchases—up to a maximum rebate of $500.

Generic drug prices may vary slightly regionally among Costco stores due to availability of generic supplies; however, the brand-name drugs have fairly uniform pricing. Costco's prices for pharmaceuticals are based on its *acquisition price,* the price paid for the drug, not the higher AWP (average wholesale price). Costco's guideline for pricing products is based on a percentage over its acquisition costs, so drugs are frequently priced more cheaply there than elsewhere. An article published in *Fortune* magazine on November 10, 2003, "The Only Company Wal-Mart Fears," stated that the markup is capped at 14 percent.

If you have health insurance that covers prescription drugs, see if a mail-order program is available. These programs are usually administered by the large pharmacy benefit management companies, and will often dispense a 90-day supply of medication as opposed to a 30-day supply. As noted before, you will generally pay less for a larger quantity of medications so the savings can be considerable—plus you won't have to wait in line to have your prescription filled or pay a monthly pharmacy dispensing fee.

KEEPING DRUGS BEYOND THEIR EXPIRATION DATE

When you buy medications in bulk, you may inadvertently keep drugs in your home that have gone beyond their expiration date. What are the risks of taking drugs after the expiration date? The October 28, 2002, issue of *The Medical Letter on Drugs and Therapeutics* gives an excellent overview that explains why taking many drugs past their expiration date may be safer than generally acknowledged. This can be accessed as a PDF file from the *Medical Letter* website, www.medletter.com/freedocs/expdrugs.pdf. Due to liability concerns, physicians, pharmacists, and pharmaceutical companies will not recommend taking drugs past the expiration date. Nonetheless, the only recorded case of harm occurring from taking expired medication is a 1963 report of kidney damage from taking expired tetracycline.

Moreover, the Department of Defense has tested the shelf life of its drugs stored in military facilities to determine how frequently its stockpiles of drugs need to be replenished. The drugs tested included ciprofloxacin (Cipro®), used to treat anthrax and other infections, and diazepam (Valium®), used to treat seizures. It found that many drugs retained 90 percent of their potency for five years or more beyond the expiration date. These drugs were kept in a temperature-controlled warehouse protected from heat and humidity, unlike the bathroom, where most people store their medications. The bathroom is perhaps the worst place to keep your medications, since extremes in the storage temperature or humidity may lead to early degradation. Both liquid and injectable drugs lose their effectiveness faster than do tablet drugs. Ophthalmic solutions may be more easily contaminated with germs after the expiration date.

Buying Drugs from Abroad

As I write this, the importation of prescription drugs from Canada and from other countries is illegal, and I do not encourage readers or my patients to obtain their medication from abroad. But a political groundswell to allow importation is sweeping the United States, and the law may be changed to allow importation by the time you read this. In Canada a different political movement is under way. Canada's health minister has proposed legislation that would effectively ban Canadian pharmacies from selling prescription drugs to U.S. citizens. Whatever the circumstance are when you read these words, the discussion of drug importation is likely to continue for years.

Many people argue that Canada is a major trading partner of the United States and U.S. citizens should have the same legal right to purchase prescription drugs from Canada as they have to purchase other consumer products. Let's review the pros and cons of importation before you reach your conclusion.

The motivation behind legalizing importation is the dramatic savings available by purchasing some brand-name drugs in Canada. So many American citizens are making online purchases of pharmaceuticals from Canada that an estimated $1 billion worth of pharmaceuticals were shipped from Canada to the United States in 2004. Most of the commonly prescribed U.S. drugs are available from Canadian pharmacies.

The largest potential savings are for newer, expensive brand-name drugs. Many brand-name pharmaceuticals are less expensive in Canada due to price regulation by the Canadian government, reduced litigation risk, and the lower per capita income of Canadian citizens. However, some generic medications are similarly priced or even more expensive in Canada.

Safety is the reason cited most often for blocking the importation of prescription drugs. The U.S. Food and Drug Administration (FDA) acts to ensure and protect the public health by closely regulating the manufacturing and distribution of medications. Drugs available for sale in the United States are manufactured in a "closed system" in which the FDA oversees the manufacturing, shipping, and storage process. Although there are no reported cases of death caused by taking an imported counterfeit drug, by taking medications from another country you circumvent the closed system and introduce potential dangers from counterfeit medications.

Pharmaceutical companies in other countries might not use adequate safety measures when manufacturing medications. Their drugs might be contaminated or counterfeit. The packing or storage might be inadequate. My patients have purchased medications from pharmacies in different countries, including Canada, Mexico, and several western European countries. Only one of my patients suffered a problem by taking a medication purchased outside the United States: she developed a serious heart rhythm problem after taking a medication purchased at a Mexican pharmacy, presumably because the medication she took did not contain the correct active ingredients. I stopped the medication, enrolled her in a pharmaceutical assistance program—these programs are discussed in Strategy 7—and after she restarted her prescription medication, she did well with restoration of a normal rhythm.

In addition, if you purchase medications from other countries, pharmacists are not available to discuss the medication with you. Canadian pharmaceutical societies discourage selling medications to patients in the United States for this reason. The Canadian Medical Association also objects to Canadian physicians writing prescriptions on patients not examined.

As discussed in the Introduction, some states are helping their residents import prescription drugs; some private organizations are also assisting their members to obtain safe drugs from reputable Canadian pharmacies at discounted prices. The Minnesota Senior Federation, for example, has developed a program to import drugs from Canada. This organization negotiated discounted pharmaceutical prices for its members with pharmacies in Toronto and Calgary. To combat this practice, the major drug companies have greatly reduced their supply of pharmaceuticals to Canadian pharmacies. The Minnesota Senior Federation is participating in a class action lawsuit against major drug companies, filed in May 2004, which argues that this practice is illegal. The lawsuit alleges that there is no law against individuals purchasing prescription drugs from Canada for their own use, so by limiting supplies to the Canadian pharmacies selling to U.S. consumers, the drug companies are acting to restrict trade.

Buying Medications on the Internet

If you decide to purchase some of your medications online, you need to make sure that the pharmacy selling you the medications is reputable. The FDA's website, www.fda.gov/oc/buyonline/default.htm, discusses using online pharmacies. Consumers who suspect that a site is illegal should report it to the FDA. Here are the tips it offers to consumers who buy health products online:

- Check with the National Association of Boards of Pharmacy (www.nabp.net, 847-391-4406) to determine whether a website is a licensed pharmacy in good standing.
- Don't buy from sites that offer to prescribe a prescription drug for the first time without a physical exam, sell a prescription drug without a prescription, or sell drugs not approved by the FDA.
- Don't do business with sites that have no access to a registered pharmacist to answer questions.
- Avoid sites that do not identify with whom you are dealing and do not provide a U.S. address and phone number to contact if there's a problem.
- Look for easy-to-find and -understand privacy and security policies. Don't provide any personally identifiable information (such as your Social Security number, credit card number, or health history) unless you are confident that the site will protect them. Make sure the site will not share your information with others without your permission.
- Don't purchase from foreign websites at this time because it is generally illegal to import the drugs, the risks are greater, and there is very little the U.S. government can do if you get ripped off.
- Beware of sites that advertise a "new cure" for a serious disorder or a quick cure-all for a wide range of ailments.
- Be careful of sites that use impressive-sounding terminology to disguise a lack of good science or that claim that the government, the medical profession, or research scientists have conspired to suppress a product.

- Steer clear of sites that included undocumented case histories claiming "amazing" results.
- Talk to your health care professional before using any medication for the first time.

The National Association of Boards of Pharmacy (NABP) is a professional association that represents the state boards of pharmacy throughout the United States. On its website, www.nabp.net, it has published a list of drugs that are susceptible to adulteration. The list includes best-selling drugs (Lipitor®, Zocor®, and Zyprexa®), injectable drugs (Epogen®, Neupogen®, and Rocephin®), and drugs used to treat HIV infections (Combivir®, Viracept®, and Zerit®).

The NABP also tracks whether a website represents a licensed pharmacy in good standing. In 1999, it developed a certification process known as Verified Internet Pharmacy Practice Sites (VIPPS™). To be able to display the VIPPS™ symbol on its website, the pharmacy must comply with the licensing requirements and inspections requirements of each state to which it dispenses. It must also complete a detailed application outlining its policies and procedures, particularly those dealing with authenticating prescriptions and maintaining patients' privacy. Free telephone consultation with a pharmacist must be provided. The pharmacy undergoes an inspection by the VIPPS™ team. The NABP lists certified pharmacies online at www.nabp.net/vipps/consumer/search.asp. The organization may also be contacted by telephoning 847-698-6227.

Given the current conditions, buying prescription drugs online from an unknown U.S. or Canadian pharmacy that has not achieved any certification should be avoided. I don't recommend it. If you decide to purchase drugs from an online pharmacy, use a certified online pharmacy such as FamlyMeds.com or Drugstore.com, protect yourself by joining the Minnesota Senior Federation, or use a state sponsored program such as I-SaveRX. While it is reasonable to believe that medications purchased in a reputable Canadian pharmacy are safe, the risk of buying and taking counterfeit drugs from an unverified vendor is real. Given the multiple ways in which unscrupulous people prey on the unaware on the Internet, it is highly likely that counterfeit prescription drugs are being sold.

To recap, begin your smart shopping by checking independent pharmacies as well as the national chains, the major discount retailers, and grocery stores to find the best price. Consider buying your drugs from a reputable internet pharmacy. Buying frequently used medications in larger quantities saves money and the time spent going for refills. Because prescription drugs are a recurring purchase, small savings add up quickly. If you are like me, you'll drive a little farther to buy your gasoline from a station charging even a few cents less. Consider doing the same with your prescription drug purchases, and your savings will multiply.

STRATEGY 3

BUY GENERIC MEDICATIONS

WHO WANTS TO PAY MORE for an identical product? Nowadays it is hard to remember the time when gas was branded and advertisers claimed that one brand of 87-octane gasoline was superior to another brand. Consumers now know that 87-octane gasoline is generic—that essentially any gasoline with that label is equivalent to the others. So we search for the best price among equivalent products and work a little harder to find a bargain.

Pharmaceutical companies examine many chemicals, looking for those containing active ingredients to treat illnesses. Each successful active ingredient that becomes a marketed drug receives two names. One is the generic name; the other is the brand name under which the drug is advertised. Pharmaceutical companies spend billions of dollars annually promoting their brand-name medications. The drug and its effects under either name are identical. Substituting a generic for a brand-name drug is a great way to save money, particularly when the drug becomes available without a prescription. Then you can save up to 90 percent off of the original price.

Don't be confused by the difference between over-the-counter drugs and generic drugs. An over-the-counter drug is available without a prescription at pharmacies and other retailers; a generic drug is a copy of a brand-name drug. Many brand-name drugs, including Zantac®, Claritin®, and Motrin®, were initially available by prescription but are now available over-the-counter at many retailers and pharmacies. The FDA has decided that these drugs are safe to take in certain (usually relatively low) doses without a doctor's supervision and direction.

Generics version of these drugs—ranitidine for Zantac®, loratadine for Claritin®, and ibuprofen for Motrin®—are also available in the same doses as over-the-counter drugs. In addition, prescription-strength Zantac® and Motrin®, as well as their prescription-strength generic substitutes, are available at pharmacies with a doctor's prescription.

Medication Patents

Patents protect the pharmaceutical companies' investments, including their costs of research, development, marketing, and promotion. A patent gives one company the exclusive right to sell a drug for twenty years and prohibits other manufacturers from selling the same drug at a discount. During the time that a popular brand-name medication is receiving patent protection, other drug companies will frequently manufacture a similar chemical, patent and brand the chemical, then sell it as a rival to the original medication. After a drug's patent expires, companies can introduce competitive generic versions of the drug.

Brand-name drugs sold in the United States produce the bulk of income for pharmaceutical companies. In order to extend the period of profitability, manufacturers try many tactics to delay expiration of the patent, such as changing the composition of the tablet coating to make a drug longer-acting. Once a drug goes off patent, sales drop and earnings decrease significantly. Schering-Plough HealthCare Products' loss of patent protection for Claritin®, coupled with the development of generic loratadine, is a recent example.

Schering fought hard to have the patent extended on its most profitable drug, Claritin®. A true blockbuster medication, Claritin® was the first approved nonsedating antihistamine used to treat the effects of seasonal allergies. In 2001, U.S. sales of prescription Claritin® were $2.7 billion, about a third of the company's total revenues. The patent on Claritin® expired in late 2002, and its sales fell with the new availability of generic loratadine. Claritin®'s 2002

U.S. sales were $1.4 billion and exceeded the sales of the competing two nonsedating antihistamines, Zyrtec® and Allegra®, each with more than $1 billion in sales. Since only three pharmaceutical companies were marketing nonsedating antihistamines, other pharmaceutical companies devised strategies to enter this lucrative market.

Beginning in 2003, the FDA authorized the sale of Claritin® without a prescription, and its U.S. prescription sales plummeted to just $25 million, as Schering marketed its newer brand-name non-sedating antihistamine, Clarinex®. Concurrently, Wyeth Pharmaceuticals began selling generic loratadine, the chemical name or principal ingredient of Claritin®, under the new brand name Alavert™. Geneva Pharmaceuticals also manufactures generic loratadine, which is sold by many pharmacies as a store brand.

Savings on Generic Drugs

Prior to its patent expiration, ten 10 mg tablets of Claritin® had a retail acquisition price around $25. After the patent expiration, a local chain pharmacy priced ten 10 mg tablets of Claritin® at $9.99; fifteen 10 mg tablets of Alavert™ at $9.99; and ninety 10 mg tablets of loratadine at $19.99. The expiration of the Claritin® patent, as well as its availability without a prescription, created a new market that resulted in tremendous savings for consumers by allowing for competition.

Generic drugs cost less than brand-name drugs because generic manufacturers do not have to invest in the costs of developing a new drug or marketing a name brand. The Tufts Center for the Study of Drug Development reported that manufacturers typically spend more than $800 million to develop a new drug over a period of 10 to 15 years. More information about the process of developing new drugs is available on Tufts' website at csdd.tufts.edu/NewsEvents/RecentNews.asp?newsid=4. Since they don't incur the expensive research expenses, manufacturers of generics can profitably sell their products at substantial discounts. Once a generic drug is approved, there is competition among different manufacturers, and its price plummets.

Like other pharmaceutical companies, Schering-Plough has developed many chemicals that ultimately have not proven useful enough to become brand-name pharmaceuticals. The sales of Claritin® funded both the development of other chemicals and the dividend payments distributed to Schering-Plough shareholders. Since Schering-Plough invested millions in developing and branding Claritin®, its sales price was understandably the highest, at $9.99 for ten tablets.

Until recently, Wyeth Pharmaceuticals did not manufacture or market a nonsedating antihistamine; however, it made other popular, over-the-counter drugs, including Advil® and Robitussin®. Wyeth received approval from the FDA to manufacture loratadine and now markets the chemical under the brand name Alavert™. Since Wyeth does not have to recoup developmental costs but does have marketing expenses to recoup, the sales price of Alavert™ in the example above was less than Claritin® at $9.99 for fifteen tablets.

Geneva Pharmaceuticals, one of the largest generic pharmaceutical companies, also produces generic loratadine, which is resold as a store brand. Although you may not have heard of Geneva Pharmaceuticals, this company is able to produce more than 10 billion tablets and capsules each year. Geneva is an affiliate of Novartis, a pharmaceutical conglomerate based in Switzerland with more than $20 billion in annual sales. Since there are no developmental or marketing costs, the ninety generic loratadine tablets in our example were priced much less, at $19.99. At Costco pharmacy, 180 generic 10 mg tablets were priced at $15.99—less than a dime per tablet.

In all three cases, the chemical loratadine is produced according to FDA regulations and guidelines. Even though manufacturers of generics do not need to repeat clinical studies to demonstrate a drug's effectiveness, it is still difficult for them to receive approval to make and sell a generic drug. The FDA requires bioequivalence—that the generic drug be interchangeable with the brand-name drug under all indications.

The process for approval of a generic drug lasts an average of twenty months, with several review cycles. In 2003, 479 applications for generic drugs were submitted to the FDA and 263 generic drugs were approved; in 2004, a record 380 generic drugs were approved. The FDA also reports (in an article available at www.fda.gov/fdac/ features/2003/503_drug.html) that more than 50 percent of prescriptions filled are for generics. This percentage has increased from just 12 percent two decades ago.

The major difference between brand-name and generic drugs is price. In 2002, a consumer paid more than $2 for each tablet. In 2003, after loratadine was made available as a generic without a prescription, a consumer paid 99 cents, 67 cents, or 40 cents for each tablet. Since then the prices have continued to decrease.

Not surprisingly, insurance companies petitioned the FDA to allow the three other nonsedating antihistamines, Zyrtec®, Allegra®, and Clarinex® to be made available over-the-counter. They argue that these medications are safe and that consumers should not need a physician to prescribe them. If these medications became available without a prescription, the cost of Zyrtec®, Allegra®, and Clarinex® would be directly transferred to consumers, thus saving insurance companies hundreds of millions of dollars. Revenues earned from the sales of these medications would likely fall dramatically because consumers would buy less if they had to shoulder the whole cost directly. The drug manufacturers successfully defeated this proposal.

Generic Versus Brand-Name Drugs

The FDA carefully regulates both brand-name and generic drug manufacturers. It requires generic drugs to have the same quality, strength, purity, and stability as brand-name drugs and requires all drugs to be safe and effective. Since generic drugs use the same active ingredients and have been shown to work the same way in the body, they have the same risks and benefits as their brand-name counterparts. In the United States, trademark laws do not allow a generic drug to look exactly like the brand-name drug. Colors, flavors, and certain other inactive ingredients may also be different between brand-name and generic medications.

Generic drugs are as safe as brand-name drugs because the FDA inspects the facilities of both brand-name and generic drug manufacturers, and both must meet the same standards of good manufacturing practices. The FDA won't permit drugs to be made in substandard facilities and conducts about 3,500 inspections a year to ensure that standards are met. The FDA levies heavy fines when standards are not met. Generic drugs are produced in facilities comparable to (and sometimes the same as) those of brand-name firms. In fact, large pharmaceutical companies produce an estimated 50 percent of generic drugs in the United States, and this percentage is increasing. In February 2005, Novartis announced that it was buying two generic drug manufacturers, Heval AG and Eon Labs, for $8.3 billion. This pharmaceutic giant, which manufactures many brand-name drugs, encouraged its employees to purchase generic drugs to reduce its own health care costs.

Some consumers incorrectly believe that generic drugs are inferior to brand-name medications. In fact, generic drugs are equivalent to brand-name drugs in quality, safety, strength, dosage, and performance. More information about generic medications is available on the FDA website at www.fda.gov/cder/ogd/index.htm. Several of the most prescribed drugs in the United States are generic medications, including atenolol, furosemide, amoxicillin, hydrochlorothiazide, and hydrocodone with acetaminophen.

Not only are frequently prescribed drugs available as generics; some of the most effective drugs are generics. As briefly discussed in the first chapter, the National Institutes of Health, at a cost to taxpayers of tens of millions of dollars, enrolled more than 40,000 participants with high blood pressure to receive four different high blood pressure medications. These patients were then followed for several years to determine the best high blood pressure medication.

Generic chlorthalidone, an inexpensive diuretic, was found to be equivalent and in some ways superior to the best-selling brand-name antihypertensive medication, Norvasc®. Those treated with chlorthalidone had the same rate of heart attack or stroke as those treated with Norvasc®, but with less risk of developing heart failure. The 2003 sales of chlorthalidone were minimal compared to the 2003 sales of Norvasc®, which exceeded $4 billion. The most recent guidelines on treatment of hypertension, the Seventh Report of the Joint National Committee on Prevention, Detection, Evaluation, and Treatment of High Blood Pressure (JNC 7), state that based on multiple studies, diuretics should be used to treat most patients with hypertension. At Costco online pharmacy, one hundred tablets of generic chlorthalidone, 25 mg, costs $12.39, while one hundred tablets of brand-name Norvasc®, 5 mg, costs $138.67. More information about these current guidelines and this important study may be found at www.nhlbi.nih.gov/guidelines/hypertension/.

Other frequently prescribed generic medications used to treat elevated blood pressure include the calcium channel blockers diltiazem, verapamil, and nifedipine, which were among the most widely prescribed drugs of the 1980s. These generic medications are better known by their brand names of Cardizem®, Calan®, and Procardia®.

Heart disease is a common cause of death, and the best-studied prescription medications used to treat those with a history of heart attacks are available as generic beta-blockers. Most patients with a history of heart artery blockages should take a beta-blocker, such as the generic medications propranolol, atenolol, or metoprolol. At Costco online pharmacy, one hundred tablets of generic metoprolol tartrate costs $11.39 for the 50 mg tablets and $13.59 for the 100 mg tablets. One hundred tablets of brand-name Coreg® cost $168.69 for the 6.25 mg, 12.5 mg, and 25 mg tablets. There may be compelling reasons to choose a certain beta-blocker, such as its indications or side effects; however, you can discuss with your physician if a generic beta-blocker is appropriate for you.

Several studies in the early 1990s established the importance of a class of drugs, angiotensin-converting enzyme (ACE) inhibitors, used to treat hypertension and heart failure. Captopril, enalapril, and lisinopril have all been shown to prolong lifespan in those with weak heart muscles. The brand names of these generic medications are Capoten®, Vasotec®, and Zestril®. These generics could be considered instead of the other more expensive brand-name medications, such as brand-name Altace®, for which there is no generic substitute. At the online Costco pharmacy, one hundred tablets of generic lisinopril costs $15.69 for the 20 mg tablets and $29.99 for the 40 mg tablets. One hundred tablets of brand-name Altace® costs $131.89 for the 5 mg tablets and $165.79 for the 10 mg tablets.

Generic medications are also used to treat common ailments such as muscle pains and heartburn. Generic ibuprofen, for instance, is better known by the brand names Advil® and Motrin®. Generic naproxen is better known as Aleve®. These medications are available without a prescription and provide effective treatment at a very low cost. Similarly, the blockbuster heartburn-treating drugs of a few years ago are now available without a prescription. Billions of dollars were spent purchasing Tagamet®, Zantac®, and Pepcid®. Generic cimetidine, ranitidine, and famotidine are now available for far less money.

For example, the well-known Zantac® is the brand name of generic ranitidine. In the late 1980s, Zantac® was one of the most highly prescribed and profitable of all pharmaceuticals. Today, both brand-name Zantac® and generic ranitidine are available without prescription. The effects of brand-name Zantac® and generic ranitidine are identical; however, their prices are vastly different. Consider ranitidine an oldie but goodie—an opportunity to buy an excellent drug at a fraction of the cost of the brand-name version.

A bottle of 100 tablets of brand-name Zantac®, 300 mg, costs $385.69 at Costco online pharmacy; a bottle of 100 tablets of generic ranitidine, 300 mg, costs $28.49—a saving of more than 90 percent. Rarely can an equivalent product be purchased from the same store at such a large discount.

The following table illustrates the enormous savings you can achieve by asking your doctor to prescribe generic medications whenever possible. The table compares the prices of 100-tablet packages of brand-name and generic medication at the same dosage obtained from Costco's online pharmacy in late 2004. If the medication came as an inhaler or a cream, the same quantity for both the generic and the brand-name medications is given. In this list of more than fifty medications, the minimum saving is more than 50 percent and the average saving is more than 85 percent!

Brand Name Versus Generic Drug Prices

BRAND NAME	GENERIC NAME	DOSAGE	GENERIC PRICE	BRAND PRICE	PERCENTAGE SAVING
Antivert®	Meclizine	25 mg	$9.99	$76.59	87%
Ativan®	Lorazepam	1 mg	$16.99	$120.99	86%
Bentyl®	Dicyclomine	20 mg	$14.29	$57.69	75%
Bumex®	Bumetanide	0.5 mg	$17.59	$52.97	67%
Calan®	Verapamil	120 mg	$18.39	$103.69	81%

Brand Name Versus Generic Drug Prices cont.

BRAND NAME	GENERIC NAME	DOSAGE	GENERIC PRICE	BRAND PRICE	PERCENTAGE SAVING
Capoten®	Captopril	25 mg	$20.57	$119.49	83%
Cardizem®	Diltiazem	120 mg	$46.29	$128.39	64%
Catapres®	Clonidine	0.1 mg	$15.67	$82.97	81%
Cleocin®	Clindamycin	150 mg	$34.19	$257.89	87%
Clinoril®	Sulindac	150 mg	$22.39	$108.29	79%
Compazine®	Prochlorperazine	10 mg	$20.97	$108.89	81%
Corgard®	Nadolol	40 mg	$19.79	$187.19	89%
Coumadin®	Warfarin	5 mg	$20.69	$73.99	72%
Covera-HS®	Verapamil	180 mg	$52.69	$144.17	63%
Desyrel®	Trazodone	50 mg	$11.19	$200.69	94%
Diaßeta®	Glyburide	5 mg	$22.79	$73.99	69%
Dyazide®	Triamterene/HCTZ	37.5 mg/ 25 mg	$9.59	$66.70	86%
Elavil®	Amitriptyline	50 mg	$14.37	$88.69	84%
Flagyl®	Metronidazole	250 mg	$19.59	$236.27	92%
Glucophage®	Metformin	500 mg	$18.09	$71.99	75%
Glucotrol®	Glipizide	10 mg	$19.29	$85.87	78%
HydroDIURIL®	Hydrochlorothiazide	25 mg	$6.29	$18.09	65%
Hytrin®	Terazosin	10 mg	$25.69	$196.57	87%
Imdur®	Isosorbide mononitrate	30 mg	$17.01	$187.07	91%
Inderal®	Propranolol	40 mg	$12.67	$77.07	84%
Indocin®	Indomethacin	50 mg	$17.17	$100.77	83%

Brand Name Versus Generic Drug Prices cont.

BRAND NAME	GENERIC NAME	DOSAGE	GENERIC PRICE	BRAND PRICE	PERCENTAGE SAVING
Ismo®	Isosorbide mononitrate	20 mg	$32.89	$171.79	81%
Isordil®	Isosorbide dinitrate	10 mg	$18.09	$37.69	52%
Kenalog® cream	Triamcinolone acetonide cream	0.1%, 15 g	$8.99	$50.19	82%
Klonopin®	Clonazepam	1 mg	$18.29	$113.77	84%
Lasix®	Furosemide	40 mg	$8.59	$28.39	70%
Lodine®	Etodolac	400 mg	$69.39	$163.59	58%
Lopid®	Gemfibrozil	600 mg	$36.99	$160.69	77%
Lopressor®	Metoprolol tartrate	50 mg	$13.59	$143.99	91%
Mevacor®	Lovastatin	20 mg	$55.49	$218.39	75%
Micronase®	Glyburide	5 mg	$22.79	$93.99	76%
Minipress®	Prazosin	2 mg	$30.19	$71.49	58%
Motrin®	Ibuprofen	400 mg	$7.29	$16.47	56%
Mycolog® II cream	Triamcinolone acetonide cream/nystatin	0.1% 30 g	$14.07	$37.49	62%
Naprosyn®	Naproxen	375 mg	$18.79	$136.09	86%
Nitro-Dur® Patches	Transdermal nitroglycerin patches	0.2 mg	$65.29	$168.79	61%
Pamelor®	Nortriptyline	50 mg	$15.21	$814.89	98%
Prinivil®	Lisinopril	10 mg	$12.79	$93.37	86%
Prolixin®	Fluphenazine	10 mg	$20.99	$264.19	92%
Proventil®	Albuterol aerosol inhaler	MDI[1]	$8.55	$38.69	78%
Prozac®	Fluoxetine	10 mg	$17.82	$347.19	95%

Brand Name Versus Generic Drug Prices cont.

BRAND NAME	GENERIC NAME	DOSAGE	GENERIC PRICE	BRAND PRICE	PERCENTAGE SAVING
Reglan®	Metoclopramide	10 mg	$18.87	$107.17	82%
Restoril®	Temazepam	15 mg	$21.69	$335.29	94%
Sinemet®	Carbidopa/levodopa	25 mg/ 100 mg	$27.99	$86.69	68%
Sinequan®	Doxepin	100 mg	$24.59	$141.79	83%
Tenormin®	Atenolol	100 mg	$20.87	$189.77	89%
Valium®	Diazepam	5 mg	$8.69	$158.59	95%
Vasotec®	Enalapril	10 mg	$16.17	$107.27	85%
Ventolin®	Albuterol aerosol inhaler	MDI[1]	$8.55	$34.09	75%
Vibramycin®	Doxycycline	100 mg	$19.69	$444.99	96%
Vistaril®	Hydroxyzine	25 mg	$19.09	$114.39	83%
Voltaren®	Diclofenac	50 mg	$18.09	$180.09	90%
Xanax®	Alprazolam	0.25 mg	$12.69	$94.29	87%
Zantac®	Ranitidine	150 mg	$17.29	$212.99	92%
Zestril®	Lisinopril	10 mg	$9.49	$104.37	91%
Zovirax®	Acyclovir	200 mg	$20.52	$166.29	88%
Zyloprim®	Allopurinol	300 mg	$21.39	$111.07	81%

[1]MDI is Metered Dose Inhaler.

How to Substitute Generics

Several important generic medications are available to treat diabetes, including glipizide (Glucotrol®), glyburide (Diaßeta®), and metfomin

(Glucophage XR®). Popular generic antibiotics include cephalexin (Keflex®), amoxicillin (Amoxil® and Trimox®), and amoxicillin/ clavulanate (Augmentin®). Fluoxetine, citalopram, and paroxetine, the generic substitutes of best-selling Prozac®, Celexa®, and Paxil®, are now available for depression.

The following table offers suggestions for substituting generic medications for costly new brand-name medications. Each row lists a common ailment, a newer expensive drug, an older brand-name drug, and a generic medication. In some cases the drug's mechanism of action is identical; in other cases the mechanism of action is different. For example, omeprazole, the generic of Prilosec®, works similarly to Aciphex®, Nexium®, Prevacid®, and Protonix®; however, cimetidine, famotidine, and ranitidine work differently and are less potent. As always, consult with your physician before substituting medications. Strategy 5, "Consider Other Medications in the Same Class," will show you which drugs have similar properties. By learning about the classes of drugs you can learn how to ask your doctor if a generic drug can be substituted for other brand-name drugs.

Possible Generic Substitutes for Brand-Name Drugs

AILMENT	NEWER BRAND-NAME DRUG	ALTERNATIVE BRAND-NAME DRUG	ALTERNATIVE GENERIC DRUG
Acid reflux	Aciphex®	Tagamet®	Cimetidine
Acid reflux	Prevacid®	Pepcid®	Famotidine
Acid reflux	Protonix®	Zantac®	Ranitidine
Acid reflux	Nexium®	Prilosec®	Omeprazole
Arthritis	Bextra®	Advil®	Ibuprofen
Arthritis	Celebrex®	Naprosyn®	Naproxen
Depression	Lexapro®	Celexa®	Citalopram
Diabetes	Avandia®	Glucotrol®	Glipizide
Hypertension	Altace®	Prinivil®	Lisinopril

Possible Generic Substitutes for Brand-Name Drugs cont.			
AILMENT	NEWER BRAND-NAME DRUG	ALTERNATIVE BRAND-NAME DRUG	ALTERNATIVE GENERIC DRUG
Hypertension	Cozaar®	Capoten®	Captopril
Hypertension	Norvasc®	Hygroton®	Chlorthalidone
Rhinitis	Zyrtec®	Claritin®	Loratadine

Generic drugs have a long history of efficacy. In 400 B.C., Hippocrates discovered that an extract from willow bark contained a pain reliever and fever reducer. He unfortunately did not publicize his recipe. An English clergyman ultimately rediscovered the properties of the willow bark more than two thousand years later, in 1758.

Over the next century chemists carefully examined the willow bark for the specific chemical responsible for its properties. In 1897, Felix Hoffman, a young German chemist, synthesized acetylsalicylic acid and gave it to his father, who suffered greatly from arthritis. Pleased with his father's improvement, Felix persuaded his employer, Bayer Pharmaceutical Company, to produce the medicine it subsequently named aspirin. Introduced in 1915, it was a huge success, becoming the first blockbuster drug. After Germany was defeated in World War I, the Treaty of Versailles forced Bayer, a major German company, to give up its patent and trademark. Hundreds of millions of people have taken trillions of doses of aspirin, making it the world's most popular drug.

Aspirin reduces inflammation and fever in the body. These effects make it useful for the treatment of arthritis. Aspirin's primary role in preventing heart attacks and strokes is to make platelets less "sticky." Platelets are small particles in the bloodstream that play an important role in the clogging of heart and brain arteries thus producing heart attacks and strokes. A large study showed that aspirin also decreased the incidence of colon polyps, the precursors of colon cancer. All these benefits of generic aspirin are available at a daily cost of less than one penny.

Generic drugs are among the most important of all medications, and substituting generic drugs for brand-name drugs whenever possible is an important savings strategy. But it may not work for everyone in every case. On rare occasions, patients have told me that a particular brand-name drug worked better than the generic substitute, so make sure your doctor knows exactly what you are taking. Substituting generic for brand-name medications works in the overwhelming majority of cases, so discuss this strategy with your physician to help make your medications more affordable. The following list of more than 150 generic drugs available with and without prescription provides a useful starting point.

Generic Drugs Available With and Without a Prescription

BRAND NAME	GENERIC NAME	PRESCRIPTION REQUIRED
Accupril®	Quinapril	Yes
Accuretic®	Quinapril/HCTZ	Yes
Adalat® CC	Nifedipine	Yes
Advil®	Ibuprofen	No
Aldactone®	Spironolactone	Yes
Amoxil®	Amoxicillin	Yes
Antivert®	Meclizine	Yes
Aspirin	Aspirin	No
Atarax®	Hydroxyzine HCl	Yes
Ativan®	Lorazepam	Yes
Augmentin®	Amoxicillin/clavulanate	Yes
Aventyl®	Nortriptyline	Yes
Bactrim®	Trimethoprim/sulfamethoxazole	Yes
Benadryl®	Diphenhydramine	No*
Bentyl®	Dicyclomine	Yes
Betapace AF®	Sotalol	Yes

Generic Drugs Available with and Without a Prescription cont.

BRAND NAME	GENERIC NAME	PRESCRIPTION REQUIRED
Bumex®	Bumetanide	Yes
BuSpar®	Buspirone	Yes
Calan®	Verapamil	Yes
Capoten®	Captopril	Yes
Carafate®	Sucralfate	Yes
Cardizem®	Diltiazem	Yes
Cardura®	Doxazosin	Yes
Catapres®	Clonidine	Yes
Cefzil®	Cefprozil	Yes
Celexa®	Citalopram	Yes
Cipro®	Ciprofloxacin	Yes
Claritin®	Loratadine	No
Cleocin®	Clindamycin	Yes
Clinoril®	Sulindac	Yes
Clozaril®	Clozapine	Yes
Compazine®	Prochlorperazine	Yes
Cordarone®	Amiodarone	Yes
Corgard®	Nadolol	Yes
Coumadin®	Warfarin	Yes
Covera-HS®	Verapamil	Yes
Darvocet-N®	Propoxyphene N/acetaminophen	Yes
Deltasone®	Prednisone	Yes
Demadex®	Torsemide	Yes

Generic Drugs Available with and Without a Prescription cont.

BRAND NAME	GENERIC NAME	PRESCRIPTION REQUIRED
Desogen®	Desogestrel/ethinyl estradiol	Yes
Desyrel®	Trazodone	Yes
Diaßeta®	Glyburide	Yes
Diflucan®	Fluconazole	Yes
Dilantin®	Phenytoin	Yes
Ditropan®	Oxybutynin	Yes
Dyazide®	Triamterene/HCTZ	Yes
Elavil®	Amitriptyline	Yes
Estrace®	Estradiol	Yes
Flagyl®	Metronidazole	Yes
Flexeril®	Cyclobenzaprine	Yes
Floxin®	Ofloxacin	Yes
Glucophage®	Metformin	Yes
Glucotrol®	Glipizide	Yes
Glucovance®	Metformin/glyburide	Yes
Halcion®	Triazolam	Yes
HydroDIURIL®	Hydrochlorothiazide (HCTZ)	Yes
Hygroton®	Chlorthalidone	Yes
Hytrin®	Terazosin	Yes
Imdur®	Isosorbide mononitrate	Yes
Inderal®	Propranolol	Yes
Indocin®	Indomethacin	Yes
Ismo®	Isosorbide mononitrate	Yes

Generic Drugs Available with and Without a Prescription cont.

BRAND NAME	GENERIC NAME	PRESCRIPTION REQUIRED
Isoptin®	Verapamil	Yes
Isordil®	Isosorbide dinitrate	Yes
K-Dur®	Potassium chloride	Yes
Keflex®	Cephalexin	Yes
Kenalog® cream	Triamcinolone acetonide cream	Yes
Klonopin®	Clonazepam	Yes
Lanoxin®	Digoxin	Yes
Lasix®	Furosemide	Yes
Levothroid®	Levothyroxine	Yes
Levoxyl®	Levothyroxine	Yes
Lodine®	Etodolac	Yes
Lopid®	Gemfibrozil	Yes
Lopressor®	Metoprolol tartrate	Yes
Lotensin®	Benazepril	Yes
Lotensin HCT®	Benazepril/HCTZ	Yes
Lozol®	Indapamide	Yes
Macrobid®	Nitrofurantoin	Yes
Maxzide®	Triamterene/HCTZ	Yes
Medrol®	Methylprednisolone	Yes
Mevacor®	Lovastatin	Yes
Micro-K®	Potassium chloride	Yes
Micronase®	Glyburide	Yes
Minipress®	Prazosin	Yes

Generic Drugs Available with and Without a Prescription cont.

BRAND NAME	GENERIC NAME	PRESCRIPTION REQUIRED
Minocin®	Minocycline	Yes
Modicon®	Norethindrone/ethinyl estradiol	Yes
Monopril®	Fosinopril	Yes
Monopril HCT®	Fosinopril/HCTZ	Yes
Motrin®	Ibuprofen	No
Mycolog® II cream	Triamcinolone acetonide cream/nystatin	Yes
Mycostatin®	Nystatin	Yes
Naprosyn®	Naproxen	Yes†
Navane®	Thiothixene	Yes
Neurontin®	Gabapentin	Yes
Nitro-Dur® patches	Transdermal nitroglycerin patches	Yes
Nolvadex®	Tamoxifen	Yes
Norpace®	Disopyramide	Yes
Ortho-Cept®	Desogestrel/ethinyl estradiol	Yes
Ortho-Cyclin®	Norgestimate/ethinyl estadiol	Yes
Oxycontin®	Oxycodone	Yes
Pamelor®	Nortriptyline	Yes
Paxil®	Paroxetine	Yes
Pen-Vee K®	Penicillin VK	Yes
Pepcid®	Famotidine	No‡
Percocet®	Oxycodone/acetaminophen	Yes
Persantine®	Dipyridamole	Yes
Phenergan®	Promethazine	Yes

Generic Drugs Available with and Without a Prescription cont.

BRAND NAME	GENERIC NAME	PRESCRIPTION REQUIRED
Plendil®	Felodipine	Yes
Pletal®	Cilostazol	Yes
Prilosec®	Omeprazole	No§
Prinivil®	Lisinopril	Yes
Prinzide®	Lisinopril/HCTZ	Yes
Prolixin®	Fluphenazine	Yes
Pronestyl®	Procainamide	Yes
Proventil®	Albuterol aerosol inhalers	Yes
Provera®	Medroxyprogesterone	Yes
Prozac®	Fluoxetine	Yes
Questran®	Cholestyramine	Yes
Quinidex®	Quinidine	Yes
Rebetol®	Ribavirin	Yes
Reglan®	Metoclopramide	Yes
Remeron®	Mirtazapine	Yes
Restoril®	Temazepam	Yes
Ritalin LA®	Methylphenidate	Yes
Rythmol®	Propafenone	Yes
Sandimmune®	Cyclosporine	Yes
Septra®	Trimethoprim/sulfamethoxazole	Yes
Sinemet®	Carbidopa/levodopa	Yes
Sinequan®	Doxepin	Yes
Soma®	Carisoprodol	Yes

Generic Drugs Available with and Without a Prescription cont.

BRAND NAME	GENERIC NAME	PRESCRIPTION REQUIRED
Sumycin®	Tetracycline	Yes
Tagamet®	Cimetidine	No
Tegretol®	Carbamazepine	Yes
Tenoretic®	Atenolol/chlorthalidone	Yes
Tenormin®	Atenolol	Yes
Thorazine®	Chlorpromazine	Yes
Timoptic®	Timolol maleate ophthalmic solution	Yes
Trandate®	Labetalol	Yes
Trimox®	Amoxicillin	Yes
Triphasil®	Levonorgestrel/ethinyl estradiol	Yes
Tylenol®	Acetaminophen	No
Tylenol® with codeine	Acetaminophen with codeine	Yes
Tylox®	Acetaminophen with oxycodone	Yes
Ultram®	Tramadol	Yes
Univasc®	Moexipril	Yes
Valium®	Diazepam	Yes
Valtrex®	Valacyclovir	Yes
Vasotec®	Enalapril	Yes
Ventolin®	Albuterol aerosol inhaler	Yes
Vibramycin®	Doxycycline	Yes
Vicodin®	Hydrocodone with acetaminophen	Yes
Vistaril®	Hydroxyzine pamoate	Yes
Voltaren®	Diclofenac	Yes

Generic Drugs Available with and Without a Prescription cont.		
BRAND NAME	**GENERIC NAME**	**PRESCRIPTION REQUIRED**
Wellbutrin®	Bupropion	Yes
Xanax®	Alprazolam	Yes
Zantac®	Ranitidine	No | |
Zaroxolyn®	Metolazone	Yes
Zebeta®	Bisoprolol	Yes
Zestril®	Lisinopril	Yes
Zestoretic®	Lisinopril/HCTZ	Yes
Ziac®	Bisoprolol/HCTZ	Yes
Zovirax®	Acyclovir	Yes
Zyloprim®	Allopurinol	Yes

* Benadryl® is available without prescription for the 25 mg dosage; however, a prescription is required for the 50 mg dosage.

† Generic naproxen and brand-name Aleve® are available without prescription for the 220 mg dosage. A prescription is required for the 250 mg, 275 mg, 375 mg, 500 mg, and 550 mg doses marketed as brand-name Anaprox® DS, Naprelan®, and Naprosyn®.

‡ Pepcid® AC and Pepcid® Complete are available without prescription in 10 mg and 20 mg dosages; however, a prescription is required for the 40 mg dosage.

§ Prilosec® is available without prescription for the 20 mg dosage; however, a prescription is required for the 10 mg and 40 mg dosages.

\| \| Zantac® is available without prescription for the 75 mg dosage; however, a prescription is required for the 150 mg and 300 mg dosages.

How to Buy Generic Prescription Drugs

You'll still need to comparison shop carefully to get the best prices on your generic drugs. There is more variability in the pricing of generic drugs, since pharmacies buy from different manufacturers rather than just a single manufacturer, as is the case with brand-name drugs. Pharmacies can buy some generics at rock-bottom prices, and some don't pass along the savings. An article in the May 26, 2004, *Wall Street Journal* reported that the price paid by the customer to the pharmacy—the retail price—may be 2,000 percent greater than the acquisition price for some generics.

It is even cheaper to pay cash for a three-month supply of some generic drugs than to use your insurance at a pharmacy that requires filling one month's supply at a time. This necissitates you making three copayments and three trips for the same amount of medication.

For those with an income less than 250 percent of the federal poverty level, the Rx Outreach[SM] program is a great way to save money shopping for generic medications. Any U.S. citizen or legal resident of any age can participate in this program, sponsored by Express Scripts Specialty Distribution Services, if he or she meets the following financial guidelines:

NUMBER OF FAMILY MEMBERS IN HOUSEHOLD*	MAXIMUM INCOME IF LIVING IN THE LOWER 48 STATES OR WASHINGTON, D.C.	MAXIMUM INCOME IF LIVING IN ALASKA	MAXIMUM INCOME IF LIVING IN HAWAII
1	$23,275	$29,075	$26,750
2	$31,225	$39,025	$35,900
3	$39,175	$48,975	$45,050
4	$47,125	$58,925	$54,200
For each additional person, add	$7,950	$9,950	$9,150

* A household consists of all the persons who occupy a housing unit (house or apartment) whether they are related or not.

Those participating in the program pay only $18 for a three-month supply, or $30 for a six-month supply of over fifty generic medications. These very useful medications are frequently used to treat diabetes, high blood pressure, elevated cholesterol levels, depression, and many other conditions. To enroll in the program, you need to fill out a simple form, which can be downloaded from the program's website at www.rxoutreach.com or obtained by calling 800-769-3880. Mail the completed form, payment, and your physician's prescription to:

Rx Outreach^SM
Express Scripts Specialty Distribution Services
PO Box 63166-6536
Saint Louis, MO 63166-6536

The medication will be delivered to your home or an address of your choosing. You must submit a new application each year. Here's a listing of some of the most helpful medications available through this program for —about $1 per week.

Selected Generic Drugs Available for about $1 per Week Through Rx Outreach		
BRAND NAME	GENERIC NAME	CONDITION TREATED
Bumex®	Bumetanide	Hypertension
BuSpar®	Buspirone	Anxiety
Calan®	Verapamil	Hypertension
Capoten®	Captopril	Hypertension
Cardura®	Doxazosin	Hypertension
Catapres®	Clonidine	Hypertension
Corgard®	Nadolol	Hypertension
Deltasone®	Prednisone	Asthma
Desyrel®	Trazodone	Depression
Ditropan®	Oxybutynin	Urinary urgency
Dyazide®	Triamterene/HCTZ	Hypertension
Estrace®	Estradiol	Hot flashes
Glucophage XR®	Metformin	Diabetes
Glucotrol XL®	Glipizide	Diabetes
HydroDIURIL®	HCTZ	Hypertension
Hytrin®	Terazosin	Hypertension

Selected Generic Drugs Available for about $1 per Week Through Rx Outreach cont.

BRAND NAME	GENERIC NAME	CONDITION TREATED
Inderal®	Propranolol	Hypertension
Isoptin SR®	Verapamil	Hypertension
K-DUR®	Potassium	Potassium deficiency
Lanoxin®	Digoxin	Heart arrhythmia
Lasix®	Furosemide	Heart failure
Lopid®	Gemfibrozil	Elevated triglycerides
Lopressor®	Metoprolol tartrate	Hypertension
Lotensin®	Benazepril	Hypertension
Lotensin HCT®	Benazepril/HCTZ	Hypertension
Lozol®	Indapamide	Hypertension
Maxzide®	Triamterene/HCTZ	Hypertension
Mevacor®	Lovastatin	Elevated cholesterol
Micronase®	Glyburide	Diabetes
Microzide®	HCTZ	Hypertension
Motrin®	Ibuprofen	Arthritis
Naprosyn®	Naproxen	Arthritis
Nolvadex®	Tamoxifen	Cancer
Pamelor	Nortriptyline	Depression
Pepcid®	Famotidine	Acid reflux
Prilosec®	Omeprazole	Acid reflux
Prinivil®	Lisinopril	Hypertension
Prinzide®	Lisinopril/HCTZ	Hypertension
Proventil®	Albuterol inhaler	Asthma

Selected Generic Drugs Available for about $1 per Week Through Rx Outreach cont.

BRAND NAME	GENERIC NAME	CONDITION TREATED
Prozac®	Fluoxetine	Depression
Reglan®	Metoclopramide	Nausea
Tenoretic®	Atenolol/chlorthalidone	Hypertension
Tenormin®	Atenolol	Hypertension
Trandate®	Labetalol	Hypertension
Vasotec®	Enalapril	Hypertension
Zantac®	Ranitidine	Acid reflux
Zestoretic®	Lisinopril/HCTZ	Hypertension
Zestril®	Lisinopril	Hypertension
Zyloprim®	Allopurinol	Gout

I have found this program to be extremely useful. Almost every day, I tell a patient about how using this program can make their medications more affordable and accessible. One such patient, 82-year-old Frank, had just had a coronary artery bypass graft. He was on the following medications: Lipitor® for his elevated cholesterol level, Altace® for his weakened heart muscle, Toprol XL® for his high blood pressure, and Lasix® for his fluid retention. These are all excellent drugs; he just couldn't afford them on his limited income—altogether, his monthly expense would have exceeded $200. Using the Rx Outreach℠ program and some techniques we'll learn about in Strategy 5, I substituted generic Mevacor® (lovastatin) for Lipitor®, generic Prinivil® (lisinopril) for Altace®, and generic Lopressor® (metoprolol tartrate) for Toprol XL®. Now his monthly cost for four generic drugs is only about $24. By the way, his Lasix® was cheaper using this program, too.

STRATEGY 4

SLICE MEDICATIONS

BUY ONE, GET ONE FREE! How many times have you seen that slogan advertised by grocery stores or mass merchandisers? It exemplifies the quintessential American good deal. Years ago, when Viagra® was first introduced, some of my patients who had been happy with the 50 mg dose started asking me for the 100 mg tablets. They explained that both the 50 mg and 100 mg tablet cost about $10 each. They wanted the 100 mg dosage so that they could slice the tablet into two 50 mg parts—effectively doubling the number of doses for the same cost.

Most consumers do not realize that some medications are prepared to be sliced into two equal parts. Known as scored tablets, they have an indentation in the middle so that they may easily be cut into two equal pieces. Many other tablets that are not scored can also be sliced into two equal parts.

As we have seen, most of the cost of drugs goes into research, development, and promotional expenses. Because the manufacturing and ingredients are relatively inexpensive, different doses of a drug frequently cost the same. If you take a 40 mg daily dose of a medication and the cost of the 80 mg tablet is identical to the cost of the 40 mg tablet—as it frequently is—you can divide the 80 mg tablet into two parts and cut your cost by 50 percent. This is how you can buy one dose and get one dose free. Many drugs should not be sliced, however, and patients must consult with their physician and pharmacist before slicing medications. Some drug companies, pharmacies, and managed care plans may consider slicing medications to be inappropriate, but I do not know of any laws that prohibit pill slicing.

The Effects of Various Doses of Medications

Interestingly, doubling the dose of a drug usually does not double its effect. Lipitor®, the best-selling drug in the world, with annual sales approaching $10 billion, illustrates this point. Lipitor® is a cholesterol-lowering drug that reduces the "bad" LDL cholesterol in the body. A 10 mg dose of Lipitor® reduces LDL cholesterol by 39 percent. Doubling the Lipitor® dose to 20 mg produces a reduction of LDL cholesterol of 43 percent—only 4 percent more than the 10 mg dose! Most other medications have similar "dose response" characteristics.

DOSES OF LIPITOR® AND PERCENT LDL REDUCTION

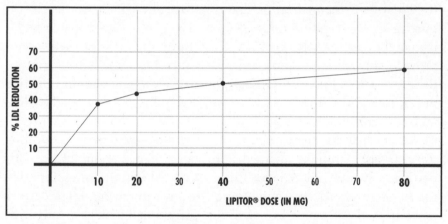

Note: Lipitor® is available only in 10, 20, 40, and 80 mg doses, shown in **bold** in the graph above.

Savings on Different Doses

Pharmaceutical companies will sometimes set flat pricing—i.e., identical pricing for different dosages—for some of their drugs in order to discourage patients from switching to a different medication due to cost concerns when a higher dosage is needed. The prices for different dosages of Lipitor® obtained in early 2005 from the Costco online pharmacy are given in the following table with a cost per 10 mg dose calculated. While the price paid for an individual 10 mg dosage varies widely, the price paid for a 20 mg, 40 mg, or 80 mg tablet is nearly identical.

Prices of Lipitor®		
DOSE	PRICE PER 100 TABLETS	PRICE PER 10 MG
10 mg	$232.07	$2.32
20 mg	$322.27	$1.61
40 mg	$323.47	$0.81
80 mg	$327.47	$0.41

Let's assume that you need a 35 percent reduction in your LDL cholesterol and are taking Lipitor®. As shown in the graph, a 10 mg dose of Lipitor® will accomplish the goal, and a higher dose of Lipitor® may be extra medication that is not required. Theoretically, if you purchased 100 Lipitor® 80 mg tablets and neatly divided each tablet into eight equal pieces, the $315.27 spent on the 80 mg tablets would provide enough medication to lower your LDL cholesterol for more than two years. From a practical point of view, you should not slice pills into eighths; however, an inexpensive pill cutter can readily slice tablets into halves.

Some thrifty patients split all of their medications. For example, 53-year-old George is a hard-driving businessman trying to keep his company afloat. George takes Toprol-XL® for hypertension, Lipitor® for his high cholesterol, and Viagra® (even though he doesn't really need it). George owns his own company, and his health insurance plan doesn't have good prescription drug benefits. Knowing that a dollar not spent on expenses, including prescription drugs, is an additional dollar in profit, George splits all of his medications.

Like other patients mentioned earlier in the chapter, he splits his 100 mg tablet of Viagra® into two pieces as well as his Lipitor® 80 mg tablet into two pieces. His Toprol-XL® 100 mg tablets are scored, so it very easy to divide them into two tablets. George effectively cuts his drug bill in half, paying for one dose and getting one dose free. He saves more than $1,000 annually by doing this, money he puts into his business or his pocket.

If you choose to slice tablets, be very careful about the dose your doctor wants you to take. Use a pill cutter with a clear cover and a V-shaped tip to allow for careful positioning of the pill in the cutter.

Medications That Should Not Be Sliced

Slicing tablets is not a useful technique for all medications. For example, some drugs use different mechanisms to delay the release of the drug so that the drug needs to be taken once daily. Many of these kinds of drugs end in CD (controlled-delivery), CR (controlled-release), ER (extended-release), LA (long-acting), SR (sustained-release), or XL (extended-release). In most cases, slicing the tablet harms the time-release mechanism and should not be done. Examples of time-released medications not suitable for slicing include the following: Cardizem CD, Effector XR, and Glocotrol XL. Generic versions of each of these medications are available in non-time-released formulations. Calan SR and Toprol-XL are among the few time-released medications that are scored and suitable for slicing. No time-released medications should be crushed or chewed.

Although slicing capsules is not practical, some authors encourage their readers to save money by opening a capsule, dividing the granules into halves, then replacing half of the granules into a new capsule. I don't advise anyone to try this technique because it is too easy to lose granules or to mismeasure them. Stick to dividing tablets.

In addition, antibiotics generally should not be split, and I do not favor slicing medications used to treat memory loss or psychosis. Some common medications that are not suitable for slicing include: Nexium®, Prilosec®, Prevacid®, Celebrex®, Altace®, Aciphex®, and sublingual nitroglycerin.

Again, be sure to discuss slicing tablets with your physician beforehand. Your doctor will know whether your medications are suitable for slicing and will need to write your prescription at a higher dose than what you are supposed to take.

Medicines That May Be Sliced			
BRAND NAME	**GENERIC NAME**	**DOSES SUITABLE FOR SLICING**	**GENERAL COMMENTS**
Accolate®	zafirlukast	10 and 20 mg	No tablets are scored.
Accupril®	quinapril	5, 10, 20, and 40 mg	Only the 5 mg tablets are scored.
Accuretic®	quinapril/HCTZ	10/12.5, 20/12.5, and 20/25 mg	All tablets are scored.

Medicines That May Be Sliced cont.

BRAND NAME	GENERIC NAME	DOSES SUITABLE FOR SLICING	GENERAL COMMENTS
Aceon®	perindopril	2, 4 and 8 mg	All tablets are scored.
Actos®	pioglitazone	15, 30, and 45 mg	No tablets are scored.
Aldactone®	spironolactone	25, 50, and 100 mg	All tablets are scored.
Allegra®	fexofenadine	30 and 60 mg	No tablets are scored. **The 180 mg tablet is time-released and is not suitable for slicing.**
Amaryl®	glimepiride	1, 2, and 4 mg	All tablets are scored.
Ambien®	zolpidem	5 and 10 mg	No tablets are scored.
Atacand®	candesartan	4, 8, 16, and 32 mg	No tablets are scored.
Atacand HCT®	candesartan/ HCTZ	16/12.5, and 32/12.5 mg	No tablets are scored.
Avalide®	irbesartan/HCTZ	150/12.5, and 300/12.5 mg	No tablets are scored.
Avandia®	rosiglitazone	2, 4, and 8 mg	No tablets are scored.
Avandamet™	rosiglitazone/ metformin	1/500, 2/500, 4/500g, 2/1000, and 4/1000 mg	No tablets are scored.
Avapro®	irbesartan	75, 150, and 300 mg	No tablets are scored.
Benicar™	olmesartan	5, 20, and 40 mg	No tablets are scored.
Benicar HCT™	olmesartan/HCTZ	20/12.5, 40/12.5, and 30/25 mg	No tablets are scored.
Bextra®	valdecoxib	10 and 20 mg	No tablets are scored.
Blocadren®	timolol	5, 10, and 20 mg	The 10 mg and 20 mg tablets are scored.

Medicines That May Be Sliced cont.

BRAND NAME	GENERIC NAME	DOSES SUITABLE FOR SLICING	GENERAL COMMENTS
Caduet®	amlodipine/ atorvastatin	5/10, 5/20, 5/40, 5/80, 10/10, 10/20, 10/40, and 10/80 mg	No tablets are scored.
Calan®	verapamil	40, 80 and 120 mg	The 80 mg and 120 mg tablets are scored. **Calan SR®** is available as 120 mg, 180 mg, and 240 mg sustained-release caplets; the 180 mg and 240 mg caplets are scored.
Capoten®	captopril	12.5, 25, 50, and 100 mg	All tablets are scored.
Cardura®	doxazosin	1, 2, 4, and 8 mg	All tablets are scored.
Catapres®	clonidine	0.1, 0.2, and 0.3 mg	All tablets are scored.
Celexa®	citalopram	10, 20, and 40 mg	The 20 mg and 40 mg tablets are scored.
Cialis®	tadalafil	5, 10, and 20 mg	No tablets are scored.
Clinoril®	sulindac	150 and 200 mg	The 200 mg tablet is scored.
Coreg®	carvedilol	3.125, 6.25, 12.5, and 25 mg	No tablets are scored.
Corgard®	nadolol	20, 40, 80, 120, and 160 mg	All tablets are scored.
Corzide®	nadolol/bendro- flumethiazide	40/5 and 80/5 mg	All tablets are scored.

Medicines That May Be Sliced cont.

BRAND NAME	GENERIC NAME	DOSES SUITABLE FOR SLICING	GENERAL COMMENTS
Coumadin®	warfarin	1, 2, 2.5, 3, 4, 5, 6, 7.5, and 10 mg	All tablets are scored. **Slicing medications used to thin the blood without careful monitoring is strongly discouraged and may lead to serious problems with the blood being too thin or too thick.**
Cozaar®	losartan	25, 50, and 100 mg	No tablets are scored.
Crestor®	rosuvastatin	5, 10, 20, and 40 mg	No tablets are scored.
Diaßeta®	glyburide	1.25, 2.5, and 5 mg	All tablets are scored.
Disalcid®	salsalate	500 and 750 mg	All tablets are scored.
Demadex®	torsemide	5, 10, 20, and 100 mg	All tablets are scored.
Detrol®	tolterodine	1, and 2 mg	**Detrol® LA is available as 2 mg and 5 mg capsules not suitable for slicing.**
Diovan®	valsartan	40, 80, 160, and 320 mg	No tablets are scored.
Diovan HCT®	valsartan/HCTZ	80/12.5, 160/12.5, and 160/25 mg	No tablets are scored.
Diuril®	chlorothiazide	250 and 500 mg	All tablets are scored.
Effexor®	venlafaxine	25, 37.5, 50, 75, and 100 mg	**All tablets are scored. Effexor XR® is available as 37.5 mg, 75 mg, and 150 mg extended-release capsules not suitable for slicing.**

Medicines That May Be Sliced cont.

BRAND NAME	GENERIC NAME	DOSES SUITABLE FOR SLICING	GENERAL COMMENTS
Glucotrol®	glipizide	5 and 10 mg	All tablets are scored. **Glucotrol XL® is available as 2.5 mg, 5 mg, and 10 mg extended-release tablets not suitable for slicing.**
Glucophage®	metformin	500, 850, and 1000 mg	No tablets are scored. **Glucophage XR® is available as 500 mg and 750 mg extended-release tablets not suitable for slicing.**
Glucovance®	glyburide/ metformin	1.25/250, 2.5/ 500, and 5/500 mg	No tablets are scored.
Glyset®	miglitol	25, 50, and 100 mg	No tablets are scored.
Halcion®	triazolam	0.125 and 0.25 mg	The 0.25 mg tablets are scored.
Hydrodiuril®	HCTZ	25 and 50 mg	All tablets are scored.
Hyzaar®	losartan/HCTZ	50/12.5 and 100/25 mg	No tablets are scored.
Imitrex®	sumatriptan	25, 50, and 100 mg	No tablets are scored.
Inderal®	propranolol	10, 20, 40, 60, and 80 mg	All tablets are scored. **Inderal® LA is available as 60 mg, 80 mg, 120 mg, and 160 mg sustained-release capsules not suitable for slicing.**

Medicines That May Be Sliced cont.

BRAND NAME	GENERIC NAME	DOSES SUITABLE FOR SLICING	GENERAL COMMENTS
Kerlone®	betaxolol	10 and 20 mg	All tablets are scored.
Lasix®	furosemide	20, 40, and 80 mg	The 40 mg tablets are scored.
Lescol®	fluvastatin	20 and 40 mg	**The 80 mg tablet is extended-release and not suitable for slicing.**
Levitra®	vardenafil	2.5, 5, 10, and 20 mg	No tablets are scored.
Levoxyl®	levothyroxine	25, 50, 75, 88, 100, 112, 125, 137, 150, 175, 200, and 300 mcg	All tablets are scored. **Slicing medications used to treat hypothyroidism without careful monitoring is discouraged.**
Lexapro®	escitalopram	10 and 20 mg	Both tablets are scored.
Lipitor®	atorvastatin	10, 20, 40, and 80 mg	No tablets are scored.
Lopressor®	metoprolol tartrate	50 and 100 mg	All tablets are scored.
Lotensin®	benazepril	5, 10, 20, and 40 mg	No tablets are scored.
Lotensin HCT®	benazepril/HCTZ	5/6.25, 10/12.5, 20/12.5, and 20/25 mg	All tablets are scored.
Mavik®	trandolapril	1, 2, and 4 mg	The 1 mg tablets are scored.
Maxzide®	triamterene/ HCTZ	37.5/25 and 75/50 mg	All tablets are scored.
Metaglip®	glipizide/ metformin	2.5/250, 2.5/500, and 5/500 mg	No tablets are scored.
Micardis®	telmisartan	20, 40, and 80 mg	No tablets are scored.
Micardis HCT®	telmisartan/HCTZ	40/12.5, and 80/12.5 mg	No tablets are scored.
Mobic®	meloxicam	7.5 and 15 mg	No tablets are scored.

Medicines That May Be Sliced cont.

BRAND NAME	GENERIC NAME	DOSES SUITABLE FOR SLICING	GENERAL COMMENTS
Monopril®	fosinopril	10, 20, 40, and 80 mg	The 10 mg tablets are scored.
Monopril® HCT	fosinopril/HCTZ	10/12.5 and 20/12.5 mg	No tablets are scored.
Neurontin®	gabapentin	600 and 800 mg	The 600 mp and 800 mg tablets are scored.The **100 mg, 300 mg, and 400 mg capsules are not suitable for slicing.**
Norvasc®	amlodipine	2.5, 5, and 10 mg	No tablets are scored.
Paxil®	paroxetine	10, 20, 30 and 40 mg	The 10 mg and 20 mg tablets are scored. **The 12.5, 25, and 37.5 mg controlled-release tablets are not suitable for slicing.**
Prandin®	repaglinide	0.5g, 1, and 2 mg	No tablets are scored.
Pravachol®	pravastatin	10, 20, 40, and 80 mg	No tablets are scored.
Precose®	acarbose	25, 50, and 100 mg	No tablets are scored.
Prinivil®	lisinopril	2.5, 5, 10, 30, and 40 mg	The 5 mg tablets are scored.
Prinzide®	lisinopril/HCTZ	10/12.5, 20/12.5, and 20/25 mg	No tablets are scored.
Remeron®	mirtazapine	15, 30, and 45 mg	The 15 mg and 30 mg tablets are scored. **Remeron® SolTab, a tablet that disintegrates quickly, is available as 15, 30, and 45 mg doses and is not suitable for slicing.**

Medicines That May Be Sliced cont.

BRAND NAME	GENERIC NAME	DOSES SUITABLE FOR SLICING	GENERAL COMMENTS
Starlix®	nateglinide	60 and 120 mg	No tablets are scored.
Synthroid®	levothyroxine	25, 50, 75, 88, 100, 112, 125, 150, 175, 200, and 300 mcg	All tablets are scored. **Slicing medications used to treat hypothyroidism without careful monitoring is discouraged.**
Tenormin®	atenolol	25, 50, and 100 mg	No tablets are scored.
Teveten®	eprosartan	400 and 600 mg	No tablets are scored.
Teveten HCT®	eprosartan/HCTZ	600/12.5 and 600/25 mg	No tablets are scored.
Toprol-XL®	metoprolol succinate	25, 50, 100, and 200 mg	All tablets are scored and may be sliced into two equal pieces. They should not be crushed or chewed.
Trandate®	labetalol	100, 200, and 300 mg	All tablets are scored.
Uniretic®	moexipril/HCTZ	7.5/12.5, 15/12.5, and 15/25 mg	All tablets are scored.
Univasc®	moexipril	7.5 and 15 mg	Both tablets are scored.
Viagra®	sildenafil	25, 50, and 100 mg	No tablets are scored.
Vaseretic®	enalapril/HCTZ	5/12.5 and 10/12.5 mg	No tablets are scored.
Vasotec®	enalapril	2.5, 5, 10, and 20 mg	The 2.5 mg and 5 mg tablets are scored.
Vytorin™	ezetimibe/ simvastatin	10/10, 10/20, 10/40, and 10/80 mg	No tablets are scored. **Slicing Vytorin™ produces a dosage different than the commonly prescribed dosages.**

Medicines That May Be Sliced cont.

BRAND NAME	GENERIC NAME	DOSES SUITABLE FOR SLICING	GENERAL COMMENTS
Xanax®	alprazolam	0.25, 0.50, 1 and 2 mg	All tablets are scored. **The 0.5 mg, 1 mg, 2 mg, and 3 mg tablets of Xanax XR® are extended-release and not suitable for slicing.**
Zaroxolyn®	metolazone	2.5, 5g, and 10 mg	No tablets are scored.
Ziac®	bisoprolol/HCTZ	2.5/6.25g, 5/6.25, and 10/6.25 mg	No tablets are scored.
Zebeta®	bisoprolol	5 and 10 mg	The 5 mg tablets are scored.
Zestoretic®	lisinopril/HCTZ	10/12.5, 20/12.5, and 20/25 mg	No tablets are scored.
Zestril®	lisinopril	2.5, 5, 10, 30, and 40 mg	No tablets are scored.
Zocor®	simvastatin	10, 20, 40, and 80 mg	No tablets are scored.
Zoloft®	sertraline	25, 50, and 100 mg	All tablets are scored.
Zomig®	zolmitriptan	2.5 and 5 mg	The 2.5 mg tablets are scored.
Zyrtec®	cetirizine	5 and 10 mg	No tablets are scored.

STRATEGY 5

CONSIDER OTHER MEDICATIONS IN THE SAME CLASS

IN STRATEGY 3, you learned how substituting a generic drug for an identical brand-name drug saves money. To save even more money by substituting similar drugs, you need to know how the medication you are taking works and which other medications work similarly. Learning the basics about how drugs work and which drugs have similar properties necessitates learning about the major drug classes.

School-age children are grouped into classes based upon their similar ages and abilities. Within the class, some have different characteristics. Some kids may be stronger or harder working. Some may play sports; others may play in the band. Drugs with similar uses or characteristics are also grouped into classes. For example, medications used to treat patients with elevated blood pressure belong to the class known as antihypertensive medications. Depending on how a drug works, it may be grouped with more similar drugs into other, smaller classes such as beta-blockers, calcium channel blockers, or other classes.

How Medications Are Classified

Many drugs work by interacting with a cellular receptor to produce a desired effect, such as lowering blood pressure or reducing stomach acid. In this "lock-and-key" model, the medication acts as the "key" inserting into the "lock" of a cellular receptor, thereby producing the desired effect within the body. Drugs activating the cellular receptors are called *agonists*. Those inactivating cellular receptors are called *antagonists, inhibitors,* or *blockers*.

Several similar drugs are able to fit into the same receptors. They work by similar mechanisms, share many characteristics, and are grouped together into a drug class. These drugs have a portion of the chemical molecule in common with one another that fits into the receptor. The other part of the drug contributes to the differences in potency, side effects, and frequency of dosing seen among different medications within a class.

In certain cases, some drugs within a class may be virtually interchangeable. In other cases, for particular patients, one choice may much better than another. For example, atenolol and metoprolol both belong to the class called beta-blockers, and both are frequently prescribed. Although they belong to the same class, atenolol and metoprolol are metabolized quite differently. The kidneys metabolize atenolol, while the liver metabolizes metoprolol. Patients with kidney failure who take atenolol can develop toxicity, as their bodies do not metabolize atenolol properly. Since the liver metabolizes metoprolol, it is a much better choice than atenolol for patients with impaired kidney function who require a beta-blocker. In other patients, either of these medications might be appropriate.

How Medications Within a Class Can Be Used

Not all medications within a drug class are used in identical ways. The FDA requires studies to prove that a medication works for a specific indication. Since newer brand-name medications receive more funding for study, these drugs frequently have more indications for use. For example, all beta-blockers are approved for the treatment of high blood pressure; however only two of the newer beta-blockers are specifically approved for the treatment of patients with congestive heart failure.

Among the older classes of drugs, such as beta-blockers and calcium channel blockers, most drugs have generic substitutes. The newer classes of medications usually have no generic substitutes available. Angiotensin receptor blockers (ARBs), for instance, are a recently developed class of blood pressure medications without generic substitutes available. Although all seven drugs within the class of ARBs are similarly priced, you might still save money by checking their prices.

The biggest savings occur when you substitute a generic drug for a brand-name drug within a class or obtain a medication through the pharmaceutical assistance programs discussed in Strategy 7. In general, there is less price variation among the members within a drug class, unless there is a generic substitute available. Learning how to substitute generic drugs for your brand-name medication can save you a lot of money. For example, my patient Henry is a 45-year-old hardworking guy who is frustrated about having to pay more than $100 monthly for Nexium® to relieve his indigestion and reflux. I explained that over-the-counter Prilosec® is a stereoisomer of Nexium®—a virtual mirror image of the compound with slightly different characteristics. These similar drugs have similar effectiveness in treating indigestion and reflux symptoms. Prilosec® was as effective as Nexium® for Henry, and he saved more than $1,000 in a year. *Consumer Reports* named Prilosec® a best buy and states that substituting Prilosec for Nexium® can save patients $2,000 annually!

Many classes have both brand-name and generic substitutes available within the class. Two widely prescribed drugs, Norvasc® and Prinivil®, used to treat people with elevated blood pressure, belong to classes with both brand-name and generic medications. Norvasc® is a calcium channel blocker. Although there is no generic substitute for Norvasc®, several other generic calcium channel blockers are available. Prinivil® is an ACE inhibitor and has a generic substitute, lisinopril. Other ACE inhibitor drugs, including the frequently prescribed Altace®, do not have generic substitutes available.

Antihistamines such as Benadryl® are useful in treating those with runny noses but have the undesirable side effect of producing drowsiness. Newer nonsedating antihistamines are also utilized to treat seasonal allergies and are among the best-selling medications. Claritin®, the all-time best-selling member of this class, is now available without prescription, and its generic substitute, loratadine, is also available without prescription. Three other brand-name nonsedating antihistamines are available only by prescription.

Classes of Medications That Should Not Be Substituted

Some classes of medications do not allow for easy substitution of one medication for another. Antineoplastic agents, powerful medications used to treat cancer, are given in specific dosages and combinations under the close supervision of an oncologist. Antiarrhythmic medications, powerful drugs used to regulate irregular heart rhythms, frequently have substantial side effects. There are several subclasses of antiarrhythmic agents, and substitution of these drugs, even of a generic medication for a brand-name drug, should be done only under a physician's careful supervision. Antifungals, and antivirals— particularly drugs used to treat patients with HIV and other infections—should not be freely substituted. AIDS drugs are given in cocktails with different drugs that work together to help prevent the virus from mutating.

Antibiotics treat different kinds of infections and are taken for short periods of time; all of which makes it more difficult to substitute within antibiotic classes. Nonetheless, there may be an effective, low-cost antibiotic available to treat your infection. When you are prescribed an antibiotic, ask your doctor if there is a cheaper effective antibiotic such as amoxicillin, trimethoprim/sulfamethoxazole, or cephalexin, available. Suggestions for saving money with specific antibiotics are given in Part II.

Different people may have dramatically different results while taking mood altering drugs such as antidepressants, antipsychotics, and antianxiety medications. As a general rule these medications should only be substituted with extreme care and careful physician follow-up.

How to Use This Section

Doctors select your medications from different drug classes for varied reasons. As previously noted, managed care companies and pharmacy benefit managers greatly influence the selection of drugs by developing formularies, lists of drugs that are readily available to HMOs' enrollees. This is done to encourage cost-effective practices as well as to decrease cost for the managed care company.

The drug classes in the list that follows were chosen because of their widespread use, as well as the potential for substituting another medication. Drug classes used to treat the common diseases of high blood pressure, diabetes, high cholesterol, arthritis, and others are presented. These classes of medications account for much of prescription drug sales in the United States.

Knowing more about your medications—how they act, why they were prescribed, and the class of drugs they belong to—will make you a more informed patient and a better consumer. Knowing when medications can be substituted within a class can save you money but should only be done after discussion with your physician. Not all medications within a given class have the same indications.

In the following pages you will find information on many different drugs, which diseases and conditions they treat, and how they work. The brand name of the drug is given along with the generic name, if a generic substitute is available. The price paid for a monthly supply of a typical drug's dosage was obtained from the Costco.com website in early 2005. If a drug was not available on that website, the price was checked on the Drugstore.com and FamilyMed.com websites. If the drug had the prices of both the brand-name and the generic substitute available, then the cheaper generic price was listed. Take only the drugs prescribed by your doctor, as only he or she is aware of the particulars of your care.

ANGIOTENSIN-CONVERTING ENZYME INHIBITORS

Angiotensin-converting enzyme inhibitors, better known as ACE inhibitors, are among the most useful medications available to treat patients with elevated blood pressure, heart disease, and diabetes. In the 1980s and 1990s, several large studies utilizing captopril, enalapril, and lisinopril proved their value in a variety of illnesses. These three medications are now available as generics and are excellent, well-tested drugs.

ACE inhibitors are very useful in treating hypertension by diminishing the body's production of angiotensin II, a powerful hormone that constricts blood vessels, thereby elevating blood pressure. ACE inhibitors reduce the production of angiotensin II by inhibiting the angiotensin-converting enzyme, an important enzyme needed to produce angiotensin. With reduced amounts of circulating angiotensin II, blood vessels dilate and blood pressure goes down.

Different members of this class of medications have different indications for use. ACE inhibitors may cause fetal injury or fetal death if taken during pregnancy. They also have other serious potential side effects that need to be discussed with your physician, including potentially worsening renal function, increasing potassium levels, or a persistent cough.

ACE Inhibitors				
BRAND NAME	GENERIC NAME	GENERIC SUBSTITUTE AVAILABLE	COMMON INDICATIONS	APPROX. MONTHLY COST
Accupril®	Quinapril	Yes	Hypertension, congestive heart failure	$38.09
Aceon®	Perindopril	No	Hypertension	$48.69
Altace®	Ramipril	No	Hypertension, congestive heart failure	$43.59
Capoten®	Captopril	Yes	Hypertension, congestive heart failure	$9.87
Lotensin®	Benazepril	Yes	Hypertension	$35.99
Mavik®	Trandolapril	No	Hypertension, congestive heart failure	$36.39
Monopril®	Fosinopril	Yes	Hypertension, congestive heart failure	$30.87
Prinivil®	Lisinopril	Yes	Hypertension, congestive heart failure	$15.87
Univasc®	Moexipril	Yes	Hypertension	$39.47
Vasotec®	Enalapril	Yes	Hypertension, congestive heart failure	$14.24
Zestril®	Lisinopril	Yes	Hypertension, congestive heart failure	$15.87

Ace Inhibitor Combinations				
BRAND NAME	**GENERIC NAME**	**GENERIC SUBSTITUTE AVAILABLE**	**COMMON INDICATIONS**	**APPROX. MONTHLY COST**
Accuretic®	Quinapril/HCTZ	Yes	Hypertension	$43.09
Capozide®	Captopril/HCTZ	Yes	Hypertension	$128.24
Lotensin HCT®	Benazepril/ HCTZ	No	Hypertension	$35.99
Lotrel®	Benazepril/ amlodipine	No	Hypertension	$66.67
Prinzide®	Lisinopril/HCTZ	Yes	Hypertension	$20.87
Tarka®	Trandolapril/ verapamil	No	Hypertension	$63.09
Uniretic®	Moexipril/HCTZ	Yes	Hypertension	$35.89
Vaseretic®	Enalapril/HCTZ	Yes	Hypertension	$69.47
Zestoretic®	Lisinopril/HCTZ	Yes	Hypertension	$20.87

ANGIOTENSIN RECEPTOR BLOCKERS

This class of medications is used to lower blood pressure. Angiotensin is a potent hormone that causes the blood vessels to constrict, thereby increasing blood pressure. Angiotensin receptor blockers (ARBs) prevent angiotensin from binding to its receptor, thus reducing blood pressure. This class of medications is well tolerated, with fewer side effects than many other classes. Unlike ACE inhibitors, ARBs do not cause cough. Like ACE inhibitors, ARBs can raise the potassium level, can affect renal function, and should not be given to pregnant women. No generic ARBs are available.

Angiotensin Receptor Blockers

BRAND NAME	GENERIC NAME	GENERIC SUBSTITUTE AVAILABLE	COMMON INDICATIONS	APPROX. MONTHLY COST
Atacand®	Candesartan	No	Hypertension	$47.57
Avapro®	Irbesartan	No	Hypertension	$48.89
Benicar™	Olmesartan	No	Hypertension	$50.29
Cozaar®	Losartan	No	Hypertension	$44.97
Diovan®	Valsartan	No	Hypertension, congestive heart failure, and intolerance of ACE inhibitors	$52.49
Micardis®	Telmisartan	No	Hypertension	$48.99
Teveten®	Eprosartan	No	Hypertension	$46.39

Angiotensin Receptor Blockers Combinations

BRAND NAME	GENERIC NAME	GENERIC SUBSTITUTE AVAILABLE	COMMON INDICATIONS	APPROX. MONTHLY COST
Atacand HCT®	Candesartan/ HCTZ	No	Hypertension	$64.67
Avalide®	Irbesartan/HCTZ	No	Hypertension	$63.79
Benicar HCT™	Olmesartan/ HCTZ	No	Hypertension	$55.09
Hyzaar®	Losartan/HCTZ	No	Hypertension	$45.47
Diovan HCT®	Valsartan/ HCTZ	No	Hypertension	$64.89
Micardis HCT®	Telmisartan/ HCTZ	No	Hypertension	$58.39
Teveten HCT®	Eprosartan/ HCTZ	No	Hypertension	$46.39

ANTIDEPRESSANTS

Patients taking antidepressant drugs require careful monitoring for worsening symptoms particularly after beginning a drug, changing the dose of a drug, or changing from one drug to another. Only physicians with expertise in treating depression and knowledge of antidepressant drugs and their side effects should substitute one antidepressant drug for another. Antidepressants are among the most frequently prescribed medications and several in this class are among the best-selling drugs in the world. Older antidepressants, particularly the monoamine oxidase inhibitor drugs, Nardil® (phenelzine) and Parnate® (tranylcypromine), have substantial side effects, have multiple drug interactions, and are seldom prescribed. Tricyclic antidepressants can cause problems in patients with certain kinds of heart conditions and are now prescribed much less frequently than newer drugs.

Prozac® (fluoxetine) was the first blockbuster of the selective serotonin reuptake inhibitors (SSRIs), a class of antidepressants with better efficacy and fewer side effects than the older drugs. These drugs raise the brain's level of serotonin (an important neurotransmitter that regulates mood) and are prescribed for many additional indications, including premenstrual dysphoric disorder, social anxiety disorder, and post-traumatic stress syndrome. Other antidepressants work by altering the brain's norepinephrine and dopamine levels, among other mechanisms. **Again, only a physician who specializes in depression and is knowledgeable about the particulars of your care should prescribe antidepressant medications. Do not change your medications without consulting your health care providers.**

Antidepressants (Selective Serotonin Reuptake Inhibitors)

BRAND NAME	GENERIC NAME	GENERIC SUBSTITUTE AVAILABLE	COMMON INDICATIONS	APPROX. MONTHLY COST
Celexa®	citalopram	Yes	Depression	$73.99
Lexapro™	escitalopram	No	Depression	$73.69

Paxil®	paroxetine	Yes	Depression	$69.87
Prozac®	fluoxetine	Yes	Depression	$8.91
Zoloft®	sertraline	No	Depression	$76.57

Antidepressants (Tricyclic Antidepressants)

BRAND NAME	GENERIC NAME	GENERIC SUBSTITUTE AVAILABLE	COMMON INDICATIONS	APPROX. MONTHLY COST
Elavil®	amitriptyline	Yes	Depression	$8.77
Pamelor®	nortriptyline	Yes	Depression	$9.27
Sinequan®	doxepin	Yes	Depression	$8.29

Antidepressants (Miscellaneous)

BRAND NAME	GENERIC NAME	GENERIC SUBSTITUTE AVAILABLE	COMMON INDICATIONS	APPROX. MONTHLY COST
Cymbalta®	duloxetine	No	Depression	$95.99
Desyrel®	trazodone	Yes	Depression	$9.81
Effexor XR®	venlafaxine	No	Depression	$89.67
Remeron®	mirtazapine	Yes	Depression	$89.69
Wellbutrin®	bupropion	Yes	Depression	$20.15

BETA-BLOCKERS

This class of medications is used to lower blood pressure. Beta-blockers are frequently given to patients with blockages in the coronary arteries or a weak heart muscle. Upon physical activity or emotional stress, the body secretes the stress hormones epinephrine and norepinephrine, which bind to alpha- and beta-receptors. Stimulation of these receptors makes the blood pressure rise and the heart race. By blocking the beta-receptors, the effects of adrenaline are diminished, causing a lowering of the blood pressure and slowing of the pulse. Two drugs, Coreg® and Trandate®, work a little differently as they block alpha-receptors as well as beta-receptors, thus dilating the blood vessels. Sectral® and Visken® have a property known as intrinsic sympathomimetic activity which keeps the heart rate from slowing as much as with other beta-blockers.

Beta-Blockers

BRAND NAME	GENERIC NAME	GENERIC SUBSTITUTE AVAILABLE	COMMON INDICATIONS	APPROX. MONTHLY COST
Blocadren®	Timolol	Yes	Hypertension	$17.87
Coreg®	Carvedilol	No	Hypertension, congestive heart failure	$101.27
Corgard®	Nadolol	Yes	Hypertension	$15.39
Inderal®	Propranolol	Yes	Hypertension	$12.87
Kerlone®	Betaxolol	Yes	Hypertension	$24.87
Lopressor®	Metoprolol tartrate	Yes	Hypertension	$8.87
Sectral®	Acebutolol	Yes	Hypertension	$14.40
Tenormin®	Atenolol	Yes	Hypertension	$6.67
Toprol-XL®	Metoprolol succinate	No	Hypertension, congestive heart failure	$34.99
Trandate®	Labetalol	Yes	Hypertension	$25.25
Visken®	Pindolol	Yes	Hypertension	$6.87
Zebeta®	Bisoprolol	Yes	Hypertension	$31.87

Beta-Blocker Combinations				
BRAND NAME	**GENERIC NAME**	**GENERIC SUBSTITUTE AVAILABLE**	**COMMON INDICATIONS**	**APPROX. MONTHLY COST**
Corzide®	Nadolol/bendro-flumethiazide	No	Hypertension	$78.39
Tenoretic®	Atenolol/HCTZ	Yes	Hypertension	$45.99
Timolide®	Timolol/HCTZ	No	Hypertension	$24.87
Ziac®	Bisoprolol/HCTZ	Yes	Hypertension	$47.39

CALCIUM CHANNEL RECEPTOR BLOCKERS

These medications lower blood pressure by diminishing the flow of calcium across channels in blood vessels and in the heart muscle. There are three major subclasses of calcium channel blockers. The first subclass, dihydropyridine calcium channel blockers, lower blood pressure by dilating the blood vessels *without* slowing the heart rate. The other subclasses of calcium channel blockers, the benzothiazepines and diphenylalkylamines, slow the heart rate as well as lower the blood pressure.

Calcium Channel Blockers (Benzothiazepine Subclass)				
BRAND NAME	**GENERIC NAME**	**GENERIC SUBSTITUTE AVAILABLE**	**COMMON INDICATIONS**	**APPROX. MONTHLY COST**
Cartia XT™	Diltiazem	Yes	Hypertension	$31.09
Cardizem® CD	Diltiazem	Yes	Hypertension	$31.09
Dilacor®	Diltiazem	Yes	Hypertension	$31.09
Tiazac®	Diltiazem	Yes	Hypertension	$31.09

Calcium Channel Blockers (Dihydropyridine Subclass)

BRAND NAME	GENERIC NAME	GENERIC SUBSTITUTE AVAILABLE	COMMON INDICATIONS	APPROX. MONTHLY COST
Adalat® CC	Nifedipine	Yes	Hypertension	$42.69
Cardene®	Nicardipine	Yes	Hypertension	$31.29
DynaCirc®	Isradipine	No	Hypertension	$54.99
Norvasc®	Amlodipine	No	Hypertension	$44.97
Plendil®	Felodipine	Yes	Hypertension	$39.39
Procardia®	Nifedipine	Yes	Hypertension	$38.87
Sular®	Nisoldipine	No	Hypertension	$43.47

Calcium Channel Blockers (Diphenylalkylamine Subclass)

BRAND NAME	GENERIC NAME	GENERIC SUBSTITUTE AVAILABLE	COMMON INDICATIONS	APPROX. MONTHLY COST
Calan SR®	Verapamil	Yes	Hypertension	$16.49
Covera-HS®	Verapamil	Yes	Hypertension	$16.49
Isoptin SR®	Verapamil	Yes	Hypertension	$16.49
Verelan®	Verapamil	Yes	Hypertension	$16.49

CHOLESTEROL- AND TRIGLYCERIDE-REDUCING MEDICATIONS

Elevated blood levels of lipids (cholesterol and triglycerides) contribute to the development of heart attacks and strokes. Several different types of drugs are useful in lowering LDL (low-density lipoprotein) cholesterol levels or raising HDL (high-density lipoprotein) cholesterol levels. LDL is the "lethal" or "lousy" cholesterol that clogs arteries. HDL is the "healthy" or "helpful" cholesterol involved in removing cholesterol from the arterial walls. There are four major types of medications used to reduce cholesterol levels.

Statins, the most important type of cholesterol-lowering medications, are highly effective in reducing LDL cholesterol levels. These drugs decrease cholesterol levels by inhibiting an enzyme responsible for the production of cholesterol by the liver. The decreased synthesis of cholesterol by the liver leads to increased clearance of LDL cholesterol from the bloodstream. Six statins—Crestor®, Lescol®, Lipitor®, Mevacor®, Pravachol®, and Zocor®—are currently available. One statin, Baycol®, was removed from the U.S. market on August 8, 2001, due to an increased incidence of a severe side effect.

Fibrates are a second major type of cholesterol-lowering medication. These drugs are used primarily to lower triglyceride levels and raise HDL cholesterol levels. Although fibrates reduce LDL levels, they don't reduce them to the same degree that statins do. Lopid® and Tricor® are fibrates, and these drugs are particularly useful in treating diabetic patients with low HDL levels.

A third type of cholesterol-lowering medication lowers LDL levels by reducing the uptake of cholesterol from the gastrointestinal tract. Questran®, Whelchol®, and Zetia™ belong to this group. Although each of these medications decreases LDL cholesterol levels, each performs this function via a slightly different mechanism. Questran® and Whelchol® are bile acid sequestrants and act differently from Zetia™. Questran® is the oldest and has the most gastrointestinal side effects. Zetia™ is the newest and best tolerated.

Niacin, a fourth type of cholesterol-lowering medication, is available in a number of forms. Niacin lowers LDL levels, increases HDL levels, and lowers triglyceride levels. It is available without prescription as a vitamin, and the slow-release preparation, SloNiacin®, has fewer side effects. Niaspan®, another form of niacin available by prescription as an extended-release drug, also has fewer side effects than the immediate-release products. Any niacin preparation should be taken with food, approximately one hour after taking an aspirin, to minimize the common side effect of flushing.

Lipid-Lowering Agents (Statins)				
BRAND NAME	**GENERIC NAME**	**GENERIC SUBSTITUTE AVAILABLE**	**COMMON INDICATIONS**	**APPROX. MONTHLY COST**
Crestor®	Rosuvastatin	No	High LDL levels	$76.87
Lescol XL®	Fluvastatin	No	High LDL levels	$71.57
Lipitor®	Atorvastatin	No	High LDL levels	$98.57

Mevacor®	Lovastatin	Yes	High LDL levels	$32.99
Pravachol®	Pravastatin	No	High LDL levels	$127.77
Zocor®	Simvastatin	No	High LDL levels	$127.87

Lipid-Lowering Agents (Combination Statins)

BRAND NAME	GENERIC NAME	GENERIC SUBSTITUTE AVAILABLE	COMMON INDICATIONS	APPROX. MONTHLY COST
Advicor®	Lovastatin/ extended-release niacin	No	High LDL levels	$74.79
Caduet®	Amlodipine/ atorvastatin	No	High LDL levels, high blood pressure	$126.87
Vytorin™	Ezetimibe/ simvastatin	No	High LDL levels	$77.79

Lipid-Lowering Agents (Fibrates)

BRAND NAME	GENERIC NAME	GENERIC SUBSTITUTE AVAILABLE	COMMON INDICATIONS	APPROX. MONTHLY COST
Lopid®	Gemfibrozil	Yes	High triglyceride levels, low HDL levels	$25.42
Tricor®	Fenofibrate	No	High triglyceride levels, low HDL levels	$91.29

Lipid-Lowering Agents (Niacin)

BRAND NAME	GENERIC NAME	GENERIC SUBSTITUTE AVAILABLE	COMMON INDICATIONS	APPROX. MONTHLY COST
Niaspan®	Extended-release niacin	No*	High triglyceride levels, low HDL levels	$46.29

* Extended-release niacin is available as brand-name Niaspan®; however, generic Slo-Niacin® is available without a prescription at much less cost.

Lipid-Lowering Agents (Gastrointestinal Cholesterol Uptake Blockers)				
BRAND NAME	GENERIC NAME	GENERIC SUBSTITUTE AVAILABLE	COMMON INDICATIONS	APPROX. MONTHLY COST
Questran®	Cholestyramine	Yes	High LDL levels	$33.87
Whelchol®	Colesevelam	No	High LDL levels	$57.83
Zetia™	Ezetimibe	No	High LDL levels	$74.47

DIABETES MEDICATIONS

Diabetes occurs when the body is unable to metabolize sugar properly, causing the blood glucose level to rise. Very high levels of glucose can cause coma; chronically elevated glucose levels lead to the complications of diabetes, including heart attacks, strokes, and kidney failure. The drug bill for diabetic patients is extremely high due to the cost of the medications needed to treat diabetes, as well as the expense of treating the associated diseases. There are two types of diabetes: type 1 and type 2.

Type 1 diabetes generally occurs in childhood, is due to a lack of production of insulin, and is treated by administering insulin. Insulin is the hormone that lowers blood sugar levels by moving glucose from the bloodstream into peripheral tissues. Insulin has been synthesized using recombinant DNA technology and modified into many different forms, including Humulin® and Lantus®. The different forms of insulin have different durations of action; some have their peak action in a short period of time, while other types of insulin last for hours.

Type 2 diabetes is much more common, usually occurs in adults, and is usually due to obesity. As one becomes obese, the amount of insulin required to transport glucose from the bloodstream into tissues increases. Various drugs work in different ways. Sulfonylurea drugs and meglitinide analogues increase the secretion of insulin from the pancreas so that there is more insulin available. Thiazolidinedione drugs work by reducing insulin resistance, which makes the available insulin more effective. Alpha-glucosidase inhibitors decrease the digestion of starches so that less sugar is absorbed into the blood-stream after meals. Metformin is a commonly prescribed biguanide that decreases the production of glucose from the liver. All of these drugs are used in addition to diet and exercise in controlling blood sugars. Many patients require several different kinds of drugs, and endocrinologists are particularly skilled at combining the different medications.

Diabetes Medications (Intermediate-acting insulin)				
BRAND NAME	GENERIC NAME	GENERIC SUBSTITUTE AVAILABLE	COMMON INDICATIONS	10 ML VIAL
Humulin® L	Lente® Human Insulin [Recombinant DNA Origin] Zinc Suspension	No	Type I diabetes	$27.87
Humulin® N	NPH Human Insulin [Recombinant DNA Origin] Isophane Suspension	No	Type I diabetes	$27.87
Novolin® L	Human Insulin Zinc Suspension [Recombinant DNA Origin]	No	Type I diabetes	$23.87
Novolin® N	Human Insulin Isophane Suspension [Recombinant DNA Origin]	No	Type I diabetes	$34.87

Diabetes Medications (Intermediate- and rapid-acting insulin combinations)				
BRAND NAME	GENERIC NAME	GENERIC SUBSTITUTE AVAILABLE	COMMON INDICATIONS	10 ML VIAL
Humalog® Mix 75/25™	75% Insulin Lispro Protamine Suspension, 25% Insulin Lispro Injection [Recombinant DNA Origin]	No	Type I diabetes	$55.87

Humulin® 70/30	70% Human Insulin Isophane Suspension, 30% Human Insulin Injection [Recombinant DNA Origin]	No	Type I diabetes	$25.87
Novolin® 70/30	70% NPH human insulin isophane/ 30% human regular insulin [Recombinant DNA Origin]	No	Type I diabetes	$30.87

Diabetes Medications (Long-acting insulin)

BRAND NAME	GENERIC NAME	GENERIC SUBSTITUTE AVAILABLE	COMMON INDICATIONS	10 ML VIAL
Humulin® U Ultralente®	Human Insulin [Recombinant DNA Origin] Extended Zinc Suspension	No	Type I diabetes	$27.87
Lantus®	Insulin glargine [Recombinant DNA Origin]	No	Type I diabetes	$55.87

Diabetes Medications (Rapid-acting insulin)

BRAND NAME	GENERIC NAME	GENERIC SUBSTITUTE AVAILABLE	COMMON INDICATIONS	10 ML VIAL
Humalog®	Insulin Lispro Injection, [Recombinant DNA Origin]	No	Type I diabetes	$69.87
Humulin® R	Regular Insulin Human Injection, [Recombinant DNA Origin]	No	Type I diabetes	$28.87
Novolin® R	Regular, Human Insulin Injection, [Recombinant DNA Origin]	No	Type I diabetes	$36.87

| NovoLog® | Insulin aspart [Recombinant DNA Origin] injection | No | Type I diabetes | $67.87 |

Diabetes Medications (Alpha-Glucosidase Inhibitors)

BRAND NAME	GENERIC NAME	GENERIC SUBSTITUTE AVAILABLE	COMMON INDICATIONS	APPROX. MONTHLY COST
Glyset®	Miglitol	No	Type 2 diabetes	$58.87
Precose®	Acarbose	No	Type 2 diabetes	$59.87

Diabetes Medications (Biguanide)

BRAND NAME	GENERIC NAME	GENERIC SUBSTITUTE AVAILABLE	COMMON INDICATIONS	APPROX. MONTHLY COST
Glucophage®	Metformin	Yes	Type 2 diabetes	$13.07

Diabetes Medications (Meglitinide Analogues)

BRAND NAME	GENERIC NAME	GENERIC SUBSTITUTE AVAILABLE	COMMON INDICATIONS	APPROX. MONTHLY COST
Prandin®	Repaglinide	No	Type 2 diabetes	$79.87
Starlix®	Nateglinide	No	Type 2 diabetes	$90.87

Diabetes Medications (Sulfonylureas)

BRAND NAME	GENERIC NAME	GENERIC SUBSTITUTE AVAILABLE	COMMON INDICATIONS	APPROX. MONTHLY COST
Amaryl®	Glimepiride	No	Type 2 diabetes	$38.87
Diaßeta®	Glyburide	Yes	Type 2 diabetes	$10.57
Glucotrol®	Glipizide	Yes	Type 2 diabetes	$8.69

Micronase®	Glyburide	Yes	Type 2 diabetes	$10.57
Diabinese®	Chlorpropamide	Yes	Type 2 diabetes	$11.97

Diabetes Medications (Thiazolidinediones)

BRAND NAME	GENERIC NAME	GENERIC SUBSTITUTE AVAILABLE	COMMON INDICATIONS	APPROX. MONTHLY COST
Actos®	Pioglitazone	No	Type 2 diabetes	$156.79
Avandia®	Rosiglitazone	No	Type 2 diabetes	$85.69

Diabetes Medications (Combination Sulfonylurea/Biguanide)

BRAND NAME	GENERIC NAME	GENERIC SUBSTITUTE AVAILABLE	COMMON INDICATIONS	APPROX. MONTHLY COST
Glucovance®	Glyburide/ metformin	Yes	Type 2 diabetes	$54.87
Metaglip®	Glipizide/ metformin	Yes	Type 2 diabetes	$59.99

Diabetes Medications (Combination Thiazolidinedione/Biguanide)

BRAND NAME	GENERIC NAME	GENERIC SUBSTITUTE AVAILABLE	COMMON INDICATIONS	APPROX. MONTHLY COST
Avandamet™	Rosiglitazone/ metformin	No	Type 2 diabetes	$80.99

DIURETICS

Diuretics are among the most important of drug classes and are frequently prescribed to treat patients with hypertension or heart failure. The latest hypertension guidelines recommend that thiazide diuretics be used as initial treatment for those with uncomplicated high blood pressure. Most ACE Inhibitors and ARBs have combination tablets with diuretics available.

These drugs are used to treat elevated blood pressure and heart failure by promoting the excretion of salt and water. Diuretics work by one of three basic mechanisms of action. HydroDIURIL® and Hygroton® are thiazide diuretics that inhibit sodium transport in the distal kidney and decrease potassium levels. Dyazide®, Maxzide®, and Moduretic® are thiazide diuretics that don't reduce potassium levels. Aldactone® and Inspra™ block the aldosterone receptors and unlike the other diuretics, may increase potassium levels. Bumex®, Demadex®, and Lasix® are loop diuretics used primarily to treat patients with congestive heart failure.

Diuretics (Thiazide)

BRAND NAME	GENERIC NAME	GENERIC SUBSTITUTE AVAILABLE	COMMON INDICATIONS	APPROX. MONTHLY COST
HydroDIURIL®	HCTZ	Yes	hypertension	$8.99
Hygroton®	chlorthalidone	Yes	hypertension	$6.39

Diuretics (Combination potassium-sparing)

BRAND NAME	GENERIC NAME	GENERIC SUBSTITUTE AVAILABLE	COMMON INDICATIONS	APPROX. MONTHLY COST
Dyazide®	triamterene/HCTZ	Yes	Hypertension	$4.49
Maxzide®	triamterene/HCTZ	Yes	Hypertension	$6.87
Moduretic®	amiloride/HCTZ	Yes	Hypertension	$7.87

Diuretics (Loop)

BRAND NAME	GENERIC NAME	GENERIC SUBSTITUTE AVAILABLE	COMMON INDICATIONS	APPROX. MONTHLY COST
Bumex®	bumetanide	Yes	Congestive heart failure	$8.19
Demadex®	torsemide	Yes	Congestive heart failure	$20.87
Lasix®	furosemide	Yes	Congestive heart failure	$4.29

Diuretics (Aldosterone antagonist)				
BRAND NAME	GENERIC NAME	GENERIC SUBSTITUTE AVAILABLE	COMMON INDICATIONS	APPROX. MONTHLY COST
Aldactone®	spironolactone	Yes	Congestive heart failure	$10.89
Inspra™	eplerone	No	Congestive heart failure	$103.49

Diuretics (Miscellaneous)				
BRAND NAME	GENERIC NAME	GENERIC SUBSTITUTE AVAILABLE	COMMON INDICATIONS	APPROX. MONTHLY COST
Lozol®	indapamide	Yes	Hypertension	$30.39
Zaroxolyn®	metolazone	Yes	Congestive heart failure	$51.29

LUNG MEDICATIONS

The most common types of lung diseases—asthma, emphysema, and chronic bronchitis—present with wheezing and shortness of breath. Asthma generally begins in younger patients and presents with wheezing due to airway obstruction from constriction of the bronchioles (small airways) and inflammation. Emphysema and chronic bronchitis are diagnosed in adults, as cigarette smoking is responsible for most cases. Since emphysema and chronic bronchitis have overlapping features, patients with either of these diseases are frequently grouped together as having chronic obstructive pulmonary disease (COPD).

The unifying feature of asthma and COPD is airway constriction, although the reasons for the constriction vary among the different diseases. Similarly, some drugs are used primarily to treat asthma, emphysema, or chronic bronchitis, while others are used to treat all three diseases.

For example, beta-adrenergic agonists act to dilate the bronchioles and are important in the treatment of exacerbation of asthma or COPD. These medications activate beta$_2$-adrenergic receptors to relax the bronchial smooth muscle, thus dilating the airways. Drugs that diminish the mediators of inflammation, such as leukotriene receptor blocker medications and mast cell stabilizers, are used to treat those with asthma. Anticholinergic medications are used primarily in those with COPD. Of course, no one with lung disease should smoke. Before considering making any changes to your lung medications, you need to consult your physician.

Lung Medications (Anticholinergics)

BRAND NAME	GENERIC NAME	GENERIC SUBSTITUTE AVAILABLE	COMMON INDICATIONS	APPROX. MONTHLY COST
Atrovent®	Ipratropium	No[1]	COPD	$60.67
Spiriva®	Tiotropium	No	COPD	$114.95

1-Ipratropium is available as a generic solution for nebulizer treatments but not as a generic Metered Dose Inhaler.

Lung Medications (Beta$_2$-Adrenergic Agonists)

BRAND NAME	GENERIC NAME	GENERIC SUBSTITUTE AVAILABLE	COMMON INDICATIONS	APPROX. MONTHLY COST
Alupent®	Metaproterenol	No	Reversible bronchospasm	$32.99
Brethine®	Terbutaline	Yes	Reversible bronchospasm	$38.87
Proventil®	Albuterol	Yes	Reversible bronchospasm	$8.55
Maxair®	Pirbuterol	No	Reversible bronchospasm	$79.29
Serevent®	Salmeterol	No	Reversible bronchospasm	$97.29
Ventolin®	Albuterol	Yes	Reversible bronchospasm	$8.55
Xopenex®	Levalbuterol	No	Reversible bronchospasm	$72.29

Lung Medications (Combination Beta₂-Adrenergic Agonist and Anticholinergic)

BRAND NAME	GENERIC NAME	GENERIC SUBSTITUTE AVAILABLE	COMMON INDICATIONS	APPROX. MONTHLY COST
Combivent®	Albuterol/ ipratropium	No[1]	COPD	$67.77

1-Albutereol and ipratropium are available as a generic solution for nebulizer treatments but not as a generic Metered Dose Inhaler.

Lung Medications (Leukotriene Receptor Blockers)

BRAND NAME	GENERIC NAME	GENERIC SUBSTITUTE AVAILABLE	COMMON INDICATIONS	APPROX. MONTHLY COST
Accolate®	Zafirlukast	No	Asthma	$80.12
Singulair®	Montelukast	No	Asthma	$86.89

Lung Medications (Mast Cell Stabilizer)

BRAND NAME	GENERIC NAME	GENERIC SUBSTITUTE AVAILABLE	COMMON INDICATIONS	APPROX. MONTHLY COST
Intal®	Cromolyn	Yes	Asthma	$91.09

Lung Medications (Corticosteroid Inhalers)

BRAND NAME	GENERIC NAME	GENERIC SUBSTITUTE AVAILABLE	COMMON INDICATIONS	APPROX. MONTHLY COST
AeroBid®	Flunisolide	No	Asthma	$68.99
Azmacort®	Triamcinolone	No	Asthma	$83.49
Flovent®	Fluticasone	No	Asthma	$81.17
Pulmicort®	Budesonide	No	Asthma	$144.09

Lung Medications (Miscellaneous)				
BRAND NAME	GENERIC NAME	GENERIC SUBSTITUTE AVAILABLE	COMMON INDICATIONS	APPROX. MONTHLY COST
Uniphyl®	Theophylline	Yes	Reversible bronchospasm	$26.87
Deltasone®	Prednisone	Yes	Inflammation	$6.87

MUSCULOSKELETAL AND ARTHRITIS DRUGS (COX-2 AND NONSTEROIDAL ANTI-INFLAMMATORY INHIBITORS)

These classes of drugs are used to treat muscular pain and arthritis. The cyclooxygenase (COX) enzyme is located throughout the body. Two different forms of the cyclooxygenase enzyme exist in the body. The COX-1 enzyme is located in the stomach and kidneys. This enzyme helps protect the stomach lining and kidney function. The COX-2 enzyme is synthesized at sites of inflammation. Inhibiting the production of the COX-2 enzyme helps relieve arthritis and muscle aches. There are no generic COX-2 inhibitors available. Vioxx®, which was recalled from the market due to its association with an increased risk of heart attacks, is a COX-2 inhibitor. The safety of all COX-2 inhibitors has been called into question. This topic is discussed later, in "A Final Thought: Drug Smarts and Drug Safety."

Older nonsteroidal anti-inflammatory drugs, or NSAIDs, such as Advil® and Motrin®, inhibit both the COX-1 and COX-2 enzymes. Although these older medications diminish inflammation, they may also damage the stomach lining or worsen kidney function. Elderly patients requiring large doses of NSAIDs are particularly prone to problems. Compared to the NSAIDs, the newer COX-2 inhibitors may more selectively decrease inflammation without affecting the kidney function or stomach lining to the same degree.

COX-2 Inhibitors

BRAND NAME	GENERIC NAME	GENERIC SUBSTITUTE AVAILABLE	COMMON INDICATIONS	APPROX. MONTHLY COST
Bextra®	Valdecoxib	No	Arthritis	$90.27
Celebrex®	Celecoxib	No	Arthritis	$98.09

Nonsteroidal Anti-Inflammatory Drugs (NSAIDs)

BRAND NAME	GENERIC NAME	GENERIC SUBSTITUTE AVAILABLE	COMMON INDICATIONS	APPROX. MONTHLY COST
Clinoril®	Sulindac	Yes	Arthritis	$19.74
Disalcid®	Salsalate	Yes	Arthritis	$10.87
Dolobid®	Diflunisal	Yes	Arthritis	$21.74
Feldene®	Piroxicam	Yes	Arthritis	$6.87
Indocin®	Indomethacin	Yes	Arthritis	$10.87
Lodine®	Etodolac	Yes	Arthritis	$21.87
Mobic®	Meloxicam	No	Arthritis	$81.87
Motrin®	Ibuprofen	Yes	Arthritis	$11.69
Naprosyn®	Naproxen	Yes	Arthritis	$13.74
Voltaren®	Diclofenac	Yes	Arthritis	$19.74

Nonsedating Antihistamines

Antihistamines are used to treat seasonal allergy symptoms, including watery eyes and runny nose. Older antihistamines, such as Benadryl® (diphenhydramine), frequently cause drowsiness. Newer nonsedating antihistamines do not cause drowsiness and are among the best-selling medications. Allegra®, Clarinex®, and Zyrtec® are available only by prescription and do not have generic substitutes. Claritin® and its generic substitute loratadine are available without a prescription.

Nonsedating Antihistamines				
BRAND NAME	GENERIC NAME	GENERIC SUBSTITUTE AVAILABLE	COMMON INDICATIONS	APPROX. MONTHLY COST
Allegra®	Fexofenadine	No	Allergies	$67.29
Clarinex®	Desloratadine	No	Allergies	$65.67
Claritin®	Loratadine	Yes	Allergies	$20.33
Zyrtec®	Cetirizine	No	Allergies	$60.19

Stomach Medications

Stomach medications, those used to treat indigestion, reflux, and ulcers, are always among the top-selling drugs. The original block-buster stomach drugs of the 1980s were H_2 blockers, which inhibit the secretion of acid in the stomach by blocking the stomach's histamine receptors.

Proton pump inhibitors are newer, more potent drugs. They greatly diminish the amount of protons (acid) produced by the stomach by inhibiting the enzyme responsible for acid production. These drugs are among the most highly advertised and prescribed medications, with sales in the billions of dollars. None of the drugs except Prilosec® is available without a prescription.

If you suffer from indigestion, ask your physician if taking one of these generic, over-the-counter medications in a typical prescription dosage would be appropriate. Despite being available without prescription, all have side effects and drug interactions, so check with your physician.

H₂ Blockers

BRAND NAME	GENERIC NAME	GENERIC SUBSTITUTE AVAILABLE	COMMON INDICATIONS	APPROX. MONTHLY COST
Axid®	Nizatidine	Yes	Reflux, ulcer	$8.49
Pepcid®	Famotidine	Yes	Reflux, ulcer	$10.70
Tagamet®	Cimetidine	Yes	Reflux, ulcer	$11.87
Zantac®	Ranitidine	Yes	Reflux, ulcer	$11.87

Proton Pump Inhibitors

BRAND NAME	GENERIC NAME	GENERIC SUBSTITUTE AVAILABLE	COMMON INDICATIONS	APPROX. MONTHLY COST
Aciphex®	Rabeprazole	No	Reflux, ulcer	$123.37
Nexium®	Esomeprazole	No	Reflux, ulcer	$122.77
Prevacid®	Lansoprazole	No	Reflux, ulcer	$123.07
Prilosec®	Omeprazole	Yes	Reflux, ulcer	$24.99
Protonix®	Pantoprazole	No	Reflux, ulcer	$99.27

STRATEGY 6

PUT YOUR GOVERNMENT TO WORK FOR YOU

LTHOUGH YOU MAY FEEL as though "the taxman only taketh away," so many U.S. tax dollars are spent on purchasing prescription drugs that the U.S. government is the world's largest buyer. Each year the federal government collects around $2 trillion and spends about $500 billion on health care. This amount of money is so staggering that it exceeds the entire gross domestic product—the sum of all goods and services produced—of nearly all of the countries in the world. Two major government programs, the Veterans Health Administration and Medicaid, currently pay for prescription drugs. Beginning in 2006, the third major program, Medicare, will offer prescription drug insurance. From June 2004 through December 2005, Medicare is offering its beneficiaries savings via a drug discount card program.

In 2002, the federal government spent $257 billion on Medicare, $147 billion on Medicaid, and $22 billion on veterans' medical care. That's a total of $473 billion. States collectively spent another $100 billion on Medicaid. This chapter explains the Veterans Health Administration, Medicare, and Medicaid to help you determine if you are eligible for government programs that can decrease your cost of drugs. It also lists telephone numbers and websites for the states' Medicaid and pharmaceutical assistance programs.

Veterans Health Administration

Many veterans are covered by a benefit package that includes health care and prescription drug benefits. Benefits are based on several different eligibility criteria, and not all who have served are eligible to receive all benefits.

Veterans receiving a general or honorable discharge may apply by filling out VA Form 10-10EZ, "Application for Health Benefits," which is available by calling 877-222-8387 or via the Internet at www.va.gov/1010ez.htm. Prescription drugs are provided free to several groups of veterans including veterans with a service-connected disability; veterans receiving medications for a service-connected illness; and veterans whose annual income does not exceed the maximum VA annual rate of the VA pension.

Many other veterans are charged a $7 copayment for each 30-day or less supply of medications. For many veterans (Priority Groups 2 to 6, which includes those with service-connected disabilities rated 30 or 40 percent, those with Purple Hearts, and former POWs, among others), there is a maximum cap of $840 after which time no further copayments are collected, which serves not to impose further financial hardship on those taking many different medications each month. For veteran retirees, a physician employed by the VA must first write the prescription. I have worked with physician colleagues at the VA to obtain medications for mutual patients. Additional information about benefits is available at www1.va.gov/opa/vadocs/fedben.pdf, and information about eligibility is available at www.appc1.va.gov/health_benefits/ or by telephoning the VA Health Benefits Service Center at 877-222-VETS. Military retirees can call the Department of Defense at 800-538-9552.

Irwin is a 75-year-old patient of mine who served in the Korean War. Although he has Medicare and supplemental insurance, he learned from military friends that he was eligible to purchase his prescription drugs for a $7 copayment. Although I am "still his doc," Irwin plans to go to the VA clinic and pharmacy to get his medications filled. He is one of thousands learning how to save money on prescription drugs from information passed along by friends.

Medicare

The Medicare and Medicaid programs are more complex, and some explanation of these programs is useful. In 1965, the Social Security Act established both Medicare and Medicaid. Tens of millions of Americans are covered by these programs. The federal government has the financial responsibility for Medicare. The states and the federal government share the financial responsibility for Medicaid. The Centers for Medicare & Medicaid Services (CMS) is the federal agency that administers both Medicare and Medicaid. Detailed information about both programs is available at the CMS website, www.cms.hhs.gov.

Medicare is the largest federal health benefit program; it pays for much of the health care received by those ages 65 and older. This enormous national health insurance program provides coverage to more than 40 million Americans. Medicare covers the majority of physician and hospital expenses. Enacted many years before prescription medications were widely used, Medicare pays for limited outpatient prescription drugs, such as intravenous medications given by nephrologists and oncologists. The passage of the Medicare Prescription Drug, Improvement and Modernization Act in December 2003 greatly increases Medicare's spending on prescription drugs. Full implementation will begin in 2006 and actuaries estimate that Medicare spending for prescription drugs will rise from its current 2 percent to 28 percent of total U.S. prescription drug sales.

Currently, some Medicare beneficiaries are enrolled in a managed care program called Medicare Choice. These plans have features similar to employer-driven managed care plans and provide limited prescription drug benefits. Enrollees in Medicare Choice programs pay a copayment with each prescription up to a predetermined amount. After this limited amount of money has been spent on prescription drugs, there are no further discounts, and the member pays the full amount for any prescription drugs. This annual "cap" is frequently set at $500, and members with heart disease or diabetes often exceed that cap within in a month or two.

Many Medicare beneficiaries have supplemental insurance provided by their employer as part of a retirement benefit or purchase insurance plans to help pay for prescription drugs. These programs are frequently known as Medigap policies. The scope and usefulness of prescription drug benefits provided in these plans are quite varied. Due to changes in Medicare, the numbers of these plans will begin declining rapidly in 2006.

MEDICARE PRESCRIPTION DRUG, IMPROVEMENT AND MODERNIZATION ACT

On December 8, 2003, President Bush signed the Medicare Prescription Drug, Improvement and Modernization Act, which fundamentally changed Medicare. This complicated bill will have long ranging consequences beyond establishing a prescription drug benefit program. Detailed information can be found on the Medicare website (www.medicare.gov), the AARP website (www.aarp.org) and the Kaiser Family Foundation website (www.kff.org). Tennessee Congressman Bart Gordon provides a concise summary of this complex bill on his website at http://gordon.house.gov/HoR/TN06/Hidden+Content/Summary+of+the+Medicare+Part+D+Prescription-Drug+Benefit.htm.

The Medicare Prescription Drug, Improvement and Modernization Act created a temporary program, in effect from June 2004 through December 2005, under which Medicare recipients may receive a Medicare-Approved Drug Discount Card if they don't have Medicaid benefits in addition to their Medicare benefits (prescription drugs are already covered by Medicaid). The benefit of a discount card is available to all regardless of income and does not change any of your existing benefits or coverage. Drug discount cards are used at the pharmacy when purchasing medications, and the customer receives a discount at the time of purchase.

More than seventy sponsors offer a Medicare-Approved Drug Discount Card, including major drug chains such as Walgreens and large organizations such as AARP. The cards are optional; you do not have to obtain a card, and you can use only one discount card at a time. Cards may carry an annual fee up to $30, but some cards are free. Medicare has approved all of the cards; however, there are differences among them. Some cards are available in limited areas of the country, while other cards are available throughout the United States. Just as different pharmacies charge different prices for the same drugs, different drug cards discount different drugs, so choosing the best card for you requires careful study.

The best way for seniors to choose the best card for them is to telephone 800-MEDICARE (800-633-4227). Expect a wait of 15 minutes or more, and have a list of all your medications and dosages readily available. If you or a family member is Web savvy, go to the Medicare website at www.medicare.gov/. The site will guide you to answer detailed questions including where you live, how much is your income, and which drugs do you take.

Beware of telemarketers who call you about a great deal on a card, and never disclose your personal information to anyone you don't know. Unscrupulous crooks have stolen seniors' identities and drained their bank accounts. Although Medicare-approved drug discount card sponsors cannot solicit door-to-door or by telemarketing, they may mail flyers and hold sales presentations. If you have problems with your card that the sponsor will not remedy, call 800-633-4227 to notify Medicare.

A very useful feature of the card is that those with limited incomes can receive money to purchase medications in the form of a credit on the card. Singles with a monthly income of less than $1,047 or couples with a monthly income of less than $1,404 are eligible for an annual $600 credit on the card to help pay for medications. Despite the advertising done by Medicare, many fewer people who are eligible to receive this benefit have signed up for these cards than expected.

MEDICARE PART D AND MEDIGAP POLICIES

In 2006, the law will create Medicare Part D, a voluntary drug benefit program. Medicare beneficiaries choosing Part D coverage will pay a monthly premium of $35 beginning in 2006, corresponding to an annual premium of $420. The monthly premium is expected to increase to $58 in 2013. Those who do not join initially will have to pay a higher premium if they join later.

In addition to the premium, there is an annual deductible of $250, which the beneficiary must pay. After the first $250, Medicare will pay 75 percent of the next $2,000 cost of drugs, up to an initial coverage limit of $2,250. The individual is then responsible for *all* drug costs between $2,250 and $5,100.

For those with prescription drug costs of exactly $5,100, this corresponds to an out-of-pocket prescription drug expense of $3,600 in addition to the premium cost of $420. The $3,600 expense includes

MEDICARE PRESCRIPTION DRUG, IMPROVEMENT AND MODERNIZATION ACT HIGHLIGHTS

- Individuals with income exceeding $13,965 and couples with income exceeding $18,735 (>150% of Federal Poverty Level) will pay a monthly premium of $35 for the insurance in 2006.
- Individual pays an initial $250 deductible.
- Individual pays 25 percent of prescription drug cost of the next $2,000—between $250 and $2,250; Medicare pays for 75 percent of prescription drug cost of the next $2,000—between $250 and $2,250.
- Individual is responsible for all drug costs between $2,250 and $5,100, the "doughnut hole" in coverage.
- Above $5,100 in total drug cost ($3,600 paid by the beneficiary), Medicare pays for approximately 95 percent of additional drug expense as catastrophic coverage.

the $250 deductible plus the 25 percent copayment paid on drug expenses from $250 to $2,250 plus the $2,850 spent on the gap in coverage between $2,250 and $5,100.

This large gap in benefit coverage has been widely criticized as a flaw in the law. Defenders of the law argue that the gap makes beneficiaries sensitive to drug costs and therefore less likely to use the benefit frivolously. Catastrophic drug coverage, which is available to all Medicare Part D beneficiaries, pays for approximately 95 percent of drug expenses exceeding $5,100. The threshold for catastrophic coverage is projected to increase to $9,066 in 2013.

Individual with income between 135% and 150% of federal poverty level ($12,569 to $13,965) and assets of less than $10,000 will receive a sliding premium subsidy, a $50 deductible, and pay a 15% copayment up to the out-of-pocket limits. Those individuals with incomes below 135% of the federal poverty level ($12,568 for a single person in 2004) and assets of $6000 or less will have 100% premium subsidies, no deductibles, and $2 copayments for generic drugs and $5 for brand-name drugs up to the catastrophic limits. Dual-enrollment beneficiaries (those enrolled in both Medicare and Medicaid) whose prescription drugs are paid for by Medicaid will be covered by Medicare Part D, not Medicaid, beginning in 2006.

Individuals turning age 65 after January 1, 2006, will not be able to purchase Medigap policies if they plan to take advantage of this plan. If you are currently enrolled in Medicare with a Medigap policy covering prescription drug costs, you must decide to enroll in the Medicare Part D plan and drop your coverage or continue to pay for the Medigap policy and not enroll in Medicare Part D. If you subsequently decide to enroll in Medicare Part D at a later time, the premiums will be higher. In general, if you have a plan and can comfortably afford it, it is reasonable to keep it. What will happen, though, is the cost of the plan will greatly increase as people age and no new Medigap plans are underwritten. So you will need to think carefully about whether or not you should maintain your Medigap policy or enroll in Medicare Part D.

Currently, employer-sponsored plans are the largest source of prescription drug coverage for Medicare beneficiaries. These plans pay for a portion of the drug expenses for approximately one-fourth of Medicare beneficiaries. The new law creates federal subsidies to encourage employers to keep prescription drug coverage intact; however, there is no law prohibiting companies from discontinuing their prescription drug benefit. In general, employer-sponsored plans pick up the majority of the cost not paid by Medicare recipients. Critics of the Medicare Prescription Drug, Improvement and Modernization Act argue that companies will rapidly phase out this benefit, and ultimately many retirees will pay more out of pocket for their prescription drugs.

As mentioned previously, the VA negotiates with drug companies the price it will pay for medications and receives large discounts. Medicare sets highly regulated, discounted rates that it pays doctors and hospitals. Nonetheless, the federal government is *prohibited* by the new law from bargaining with drug companies over the prices paid for Medicare recipients' prescription drugs. Rather than using the purchasing power of the U.S. government, already the single largest buyer of prescription drugs, private companies will administer Medicare Part D.

How much will this plan cost taxpayers? When the law was signed in December 2003, the estimated expense to taxpayers over a ten-year period was estimated at less than $400 billion. The Office of Management and Budget and Medicare actuaries subsequently estimated that the expense of the program will exceed $500 billion for the first decade of implementation. In February 2005, the Center for Medicare and Medicaid estimated that the program will cost $724 billion between 2006 and 2015.

How much will you personally pay for your prescription drugs under the program? Since most of the money used to pay for the program will come out of general tax revenues, how much will we taxpayers pay for prescription drugs under the program? The following table gives several examples based upon your annual prescription drug costs. This table would not apply to those with very low incomes, Medicaid recipients, and nursing home residents. It assumes that the enrollee pays the monthly premium and required copayments. Readers interested in further calculations should visit the Kaiser Family Foundation's Medicare Drug Benefit Calculator on its website at www.kff.org/medicare/rxdrugscalculator.cfm.

| 2006 Medicare Drug Benefit Cost for Beneficiaries and Taxpayers				
TOTAL PRESCRIPTION DRUG COST	BENEFICIARY PREMIUM PAYMENTS	BENEFICIARY ADDITIONAL COPAYMENTS	TOTAL BENEFICIARY PAYMENTS	MEDICARE PART D PAYMENTS
$250.00	$420.00	$250.00	$670.00	$0
$500.00	$420.00	$312.50	$732.50	$187.50
$750.00	$420.00	$375.00	$795.00	$375.00
$810.00	$420.00	$390.00	$810.00	$420.00
$1,000.00	$420.00	$437.50	$857.50	$562.50
$1,250.00	$420.00	$500.00	$920.00	$750.00
$1,500.00	$420.00	$562.50	$812.50	$937.50
$1,750.00	$420.00	$625.00	$1,045.00	$1,125.00
$2,000.00	$420.00	$687.50	$1,107.50	$1,312.50
$2,250.00	$420.00	$750.00	$1,170.00	$1,500.00
$2,500.00	$420.00	$1,000.00	$1,420.00	$1,500.00

2006 Medicare Drug Benefit Cost for Beneficiaries and Taxpayers cont.				
TOTAL PRESCRIPTION DRUG COST	BENEFICIARY PREMIUM PAYMENTS	BENEFICIARY ADDITIONAL COPAYMENTS	TOTAL BENEFICIARY PAYMENTS	MEDICARE PART D PAYMENTS
$2,750.00	$420.00	$1,250.00	$1,670.00	$1,500.00
$3,000.00	$420.00	$1,500.00	$1,920.00	$1,500.00
$3,250.00	$420.00	$1,750.00	$2,170.00	$1,500.00
$3,500.00	$420.00	$2,000.00	$2,420.00	$1,500.00
$3,750.00	$420.00	$2,250.00	$2,670.00	$1,500.00
$4,000.00	$420.00	$2,500.00	$2,920.00	$1,500.00
$4,250.00	$420.00	$2,750.00	$3,170.00	$1,500.00
$4,500.00	$420.00	$3,000.00	$3,420.00	$1,500.00
$4,750.00	$420.00	$3,250.00	$3,670.00	$1,500.00
$5,000.00	$420.00	$3,500.00	$3,920.00	$1,500.00
$5,100.00	$420.00	$3,600.00	$4,020.00	$1,500.00
$6,000.00	$420.00	$3,645.00	$4,065.00	$2,355.00
$10,000.00	$420.00	$3,845.00	$4,265.00	$6,155.00
$20,000.00	$420.00	$4,345.00	$4,765.00	$15,655.00

By knowing how much you are currently paying for prescription drugs, you can look up your expected premiums and copayments. Once the total amount you spend on prescription drugs exceeds $5,100, Medicare will pay for nearly all additional drug costs—even if the additional costs total in excess of $20,000.

Some readers might incorrectly believe that an annual prescription drug cost of $20,000 would be rare. The Kaiser Family Foundation estimates that the average senior will have $3,160 in total drug expenses in 2006. But consider, for example, the cost of a brand-name drug widely advertised on television, erythropoietin, better known by the brand name Procrit®. A dose of Procrit® of 4,000 units—with a price per dose of about $50—given three times weekly adds up to an annual cost of just under $8,000. Patients who need Procrit® suffer from cancer, chronic renal failure, or other serious diseases that require additional medications.

Some drugs are so expensive that they may be unaffordable. Dr. Deborah Schrag wrote in the July 22, 2004, *New England Journal of Medicine* that a new drug treatment for advanced colon cancer, involving the combination of Camptosar® (irinotecan) and Erbitux® (cetuximab), will increase the pharmaceutical cost for treating this form of cancer several hundredfold. She estimates that a typical treatment course of chemotherapy would cost $161,000! Regrettably, this increased expense did not result in additional cures. Dr. Schrag then poses the difficult question: How much should society pay for treatment of advanced cancer?

So will you spend more or less money with the new Medicare Prescription Drug Law? That depends on many things. The Kaiser Family Foundation's "Estimates of Medicare Beneficiaries' Out-of-Pocket Drug Spending in 2006" (available at www.kff.org/medicare/7201.cfm) projects that the average Part D recipient will spend 37 percent less in out-of-pocket expense. It estimates that 8.7 million Part D recipients who receive low-income subsidies will benefit the most, as they will spend 83 percent less than they otherwise would have. This group includes those currently on Medicaid, in addition to 2.3 million who are not on Medicaid and who will save an average of $1,400 annually. Dual-eligibles with Medicaid and Medicare will save considerably less, as they currently pay considerably less for prescription drugs due to their Medicaid benefits.

Nearly 7 million beneficiaries will have out-of-pocket costs exceeding $750 annually (equal to $2,250 in total annual drug costs—the threshold for the "doughnut hole"), and slightly over 3 million will spend more than $3,600 per year and receive catastrophic coverage. One in four participants is projected to have higher out-of-pocket expenses, with an average increase of $492 per year. This group includes those who currently have drug coverage through employer-sponsored plans who are expected to lose that coverage.

Medicaid

Medicaid is a large and complicated government program that provides health insurance for 50 million Americans. It was initially designed to provide medical assistance to certain groups of financially needy people, including children, pregnant women, and disabled adults. Medicaid now pays for many other groups, including those living in nursing homes and patients with AIDS. Those with AIDS who are not eligible for Medicaid qualify for a different program. The Ryan White Comprehensive AIDS Resources Emergency (CARE) Act provides health care for those with AIDS and HIV disease, and more information is available at http://hab.hrsa.gov/history.htm.

With each downturn in the economy, states' revenues decline and more people become eligible for Medicaid benefits. Due to rapid growth, the combined state and federal expenditures for the Medicaid program now exceed those of Medicare. The majority of Medicaid funding is federal, but the programs are administered by individual states according to guidelines that the states develop. Since Medicaid programs vary from state to state, someone who moves from one state to another may lose or gain benefits. The Kaiser Family Foundation lists detailed information about benefits provided by the Medicaid programs of all fifty states on its website at www.statehealthfacts.kff.org/cgi-bin/healthfacts.cgi?action=compare.

Unlike Medicare, Medicaid pays for prescription drugs; however, the drugs that are available vary somewhat among states. Rising drug prices has partly fueled the dramatic increase in the Medicaid program, as it pays for many expensive medications. Annual Medicaid spending on prescription medications increased more than 16 percent from $4.8 billion in 1990 to $21 billion in 2000.

States receive money from the federal government based upon the amount of money that they contribute to Medicaid. The federal government then matches money contributed by the state on a percentage basis. States with lower per capita income receive a higher matching percentage, but all states receive at least 50 percent of their Medicaid revenue from federal revenues. In 2002, the U.S.

government paid for 57 percent of the cost of the entire Medicaid program.

States that decrease the money paid to their Medicaid beneficiaries receive fewer matching funds from the federal government. Since Medicaid is a legal entitlement program, enrollment by those who are eligible is unrestricted. Each state has some control over which services are provided; however, federal guidelines must be met for the state to receive federal funding.

Information about the Medicaid program, as well as links to individual state's programs, is available online at http://cms.hhs.gov/medicaid/. John Iglehart wrote an excellent summary about the Medicaid program in the May 22, 2003, issue of *The New England Journal of Medicine*. Much of the information in this chapter is from those sources.

The following two tables list the contact telephone number and website of each state's Medicaid program and patient assistance program, if the state has one. Disabled persons and those with small children might not realize they qualify for Medicaid. Some state, county, and city health services provide pharmaceutical assistance. Some states still offer pharmaceutical assistance programs for the elderly and disabled. The listing of states with pharmaceutical assistance programs was made from investigating several websites including NeedyMeds (www.needymends.com), RxHope (www.rxhope.com/pap_info .asp), and RxAssist (www.rxassist.org). Some states have multiple programs, but others did not have any programs listed. If your state does not have an assistance program listed, consider contacting your state representative to see if there are any programs that have not made the list. You can also research the following websites to see if there are new programs listed since this section was written:

www.familycaregiversonline.com/rx-discount-by-state.html
www.needymeds.com/indices/stateprograms.shtml
www.rxhope.com/pap_info.asp

There are many ways for you to put your government to work for you, so be sure to use these valuable services.

Where to Find Information on States' Medicaid Programs

STATE	TELEPHONE NUMBER	WEBSITE
Alabama	334-242-5000	www.medicaid.state.al.us
Alaska	800-780-9972	www.hss.state.ak.us/dhcs/medicaid
Arizona	602-417-7100	www.ahcccs.state.az.us
Arkansas	501-376-2211	www.medicaid.state.ar.us
California	916-445-6951	www.dss.cahwnet.gov
Colorado	800-221-3943	www.chcpf.state.co.us
Connecticut	860-424-4908	www.dss.state.ct.us/
Delaware	302-255-9040	www.state.de.us/dhss/
District of Columbia	202-724-5506	http://dchealth.dc.gov/about/index_maa.shtm
Florida	888-419-3456	www.fdhc.state.fl.us/Medicaid/index.shtml
Georgia	770-570-3300	www.communityhealth.state.ga.us
Hawaii	800-235-4378	www.med-quest.us/
Idaho	208-334-5747	www.healthandwelfare.idaho.gov/
Illinois	800-226-0768	www.dpaillinois.com/medical
Indiana	317-233-5596	www.in.gov/isdh/programs/programs.htm
Iowa	515-327-5121	www.dhs.state.ia.us/
Kansas	785-274-4200	www.srskansas.org/hcp/
Kentucky	502-564-2687	http://chs.ky.gov/dms/
Louisiana	225-342-5774	www.dhh.state.la.us/
Maine	207-624-7539	www.state.me.us/bms/bmshome.htm
Maryland	410-333-3020	www.dhr.state.md.us/fia/medicaid.htm

Where to Find Information on States' Medicaid Programs cont.

STATE	TELEPHONE NUMBER	WEBSITE
Massachusetts	617-210-5000	www.mass.gov/portal/index.jsp?pageID =eohhs2agencylanding&L=4&L0=Home&L1 =Government&L2=Departments+and+ Divisions&L3=MassHealth&sid=Eeohhs2
Michigan	517-241-7882	www.mdch.state.mi.us/msa/mdch_msa/ msahome.htm
Minnesota	651-297-3933	www.dhs.state.mn.us/main/groups/agency wide/documents/pub/dhs_Home_Page.hcsp
Mississippi	601-359-6050	www.dom.state.ms.us/
Missouri	573-751-3425	www.dss.mo.gov/dms/
Montana	406-444-1788	www.dphhs.state.mt.us/
Nebraska	402-471-9325	www.hhs.state.ne.us/svc/svcindex.htm
Nevada	800-992-0900	http://dhcfp.state.nv.us/
New Hampshire	603-271-4580	www.dhhs.state.nh.us/
New Jersey	609-588-2600	www.state.nj.us/humanservices/
New Mexico	505-827-3100	www.state.nm.us/hsd/mad/Index.html
New York	518-486-9057	www.health.state.ny.us/health_care/ medicaid/index.htm
North Carolina	919-855-4100	www.dhhs.state.nc.us/dma/
North Dakota	701-328-2310	www.state.nd.us/humanservices/services/ medicalserv/medicaid/
Ohio	614-728-3288	http://jfs.ohio.gov/ohp/
Oklahoma	405-522-7300	www.ohca.state.ok.us/
Oregon	503-945-5772	www.oregon.gov/dhs/healthplan/index.shtml

Where to Find Information on States' Medicaid Programs cont.

STATE	TELEPHONE NUMBER	WEBSITE
Pennsylvania	717-787-1870	www.dpw.state.pa.us/omap/dpwomap.asp
Rhode Island	401-462-1300	www.dhs.state.ri.us/
South Carolina	803-898-2500	www.dhhs.state.sc.us/
South Dakota	605-773-4678	www.state.sd.us/social/MedElig/index.htm
Tennessee	615-741-0213	www2.state.tn.us/health/
Texas	877-787-8999	www.hhsc.state.tx.us/
Utah	801-538-6155	http://health.utah.gov/medicaid/
Vermont	802-241-2800	www.dpath.state.vt.us/
Virginia	804-786-8099	www.dss.state.va.us/benefit/medicaid_coverage.html
Washington	800-562-6188	http://fortress.wa.gov/dshs/maa/
West Virginia	304-558-1700	www.wvdhhr.org/bms/
Wisconsin	608-266-1865	www.dhfs.state.wi.us/medicaid/index.htm
Wyoming	307-777-7656	http://wdhfs.state.wy.us/

Where to Find Information on States' Pharmaceutical Assistance Programs

STATE	TELEPHONE NUMBER	WEBSITE
Alabama	800-243-5463	www.ageline.net/seniorrx.htm
Alaska	907-269-3680	www.hss.state.ak.us/dsds/seniorcaresio.htm
Arizona	888-227-8315	www.rxamerica.com
Arkansas	800-950-8233	http://users.aristotle.net/~ahcaf/index.html
California	800-434-0222	www.cahealthadvocates.org/zlib/facts/A-004.doc
Colorado	None	None

Connecticut	800-423-5026	www.connpace.com
Delaware	800-996-9969	www.state.de.us/dhss/dss/dpap.html
District of Columbia	None	None
Florida	888-419-3456	www.floridahealthstat.com/silversaverdetails.shtml
Georgia	800-982-4723	www.gacares.org/
Hawaii	None	None
Idaho	None	None
Illinois	800-624-2459	www.state.il.us/aging/1rx/cbrx/cbrx-main.htm
Indiana	866-267-4679	www.state.in.us/fssa/rxprogram/rxhome.htm
Iowa	866-282-5817	www.iowapriority.org/default.asp
Kansas	800-432-3535	www.agingkansas.org/kdoa/programs/pharmassistprog.htm
Kentucky	None	None
Louisiana	None	None
Maine	866-796-2463	www.maine.gov/dhhs/beas/medbook.htm
Maryland	800-226-2142	www.dhmh.state.md.us/mma/mpap/
Massachusetts	800-243-4636	www.mass.gov/Eelders/docs/pa_factsheet.doc
Michigan	866-747-5844	www.miepic.com
Minnesota	800-657-3659	www.dhs.state.mn.us/main/groups/healthcare/documents/pub/DHS_id_006258.hcsp
Mississippi	None	None
Missouri	800-375-1406	www.dhss.mo.gov/MoSeniorRx/

Where to Find Information on States' Pharmaceutical Assistance Programs cont.		
STATE	**TELEPHONE NUMBER**	**WEBSITE**
Montana	None	None
Nebraska	None	None
Nevada	800-262-7726	www.nevadaseniorrx.com
New Hampshire	None	www.dhhs.state.nh.us/DHHS/BEAS/assist-prescription-drug.htm
New Jersey	800-792-9745	www.state.nj.us/health/seniorbenefits/paadapp.htm
New Mexico	866-244-0882	www.nmrhca.state.nm.us/spdp/default.htm
New York	800-332-3742	www.health.state.ny.us/nysdoh/epic/faq.htm
North Carolina	866-226-1388	www.ncseniorcare.com
North Dakota	None	None
Ohio	800-422-1976	www.goldenbuckeye.com/
Oklahoma	None	None
Oregon	800-762-4636	www.dhs.state.or.us/seniors/aging/spdap_info.htm
Pennsylvania	800-225-7223	www.aging.state.pa.us/aging/cwp/view.asp?a=3&Q=228861
Rhode Island	401-462-4000	www.dea.state.ri.us/
South Carolina	877-239-5277	http://southcarolina.fhsc.com/beneficiaries/silverxcard/
South Dakota	866-854-5465	www.state.sd.us/social/asa/
Tennessee	None	None
Texas	None	None
Utah	None	None

Where to Find Information on States' Pharmaceutical Assistance Programs cont.		
STATE	TELEPHONE NUMBER	WEBSITE
Vermont	800-250-8427	www.dsw.state.vt.us/Programs_Pages/Health care/vhap_pharmacy.htm
Virginia	None	None
Washington	None	None
West Virginia	304-558-3317	www.state.wv.us/seniorservices/
Wisconsin	800-657-2038	www.dhfs.state.wi.us/seniorcare/index.htm
Wyoming	None	None

STRATEGY 7

USE PHARMACEUTICAL ASSISTANCE PROGRAMS

E VEN AFTER USING THE PRIOR cost-saving recommendations, you may still find yourself needing a drug that you cannot afford. Perhaps it is a new drug without a generic substitute. Perhaps your income is too high for Medicaid or other government programs. Perhaps you suffer from a rare disease that requires very expensive drugs to treat it. There is yet another strategy available to you.

My patient Jack is a good example of someone who still could not afford a needed medication even after using the strategies we have discussed. This 50-year-old unemployed man survived a threatened heart attack and was found to have a 95 percent blockage in an important heart artery. He needed treatment with angioplasty and the placement of a drug-eluting stent. Jack was discharged from the hospital with prescriptions for medications that would cost him a total of several thousand dollars a year, including Altace®, Toprol-XL®, Zocor®, and Plavix®. Not being able to afford his medications and knowing how badly he needed them, Jack was quite depressed.

Jack mastered Strategies 1 and 2, "Learn Prices" and "Comparison Shop," better than just about anyone. Jack's sister works for a local pharmacist and was able to buy the drugs at the pharmacy's acquisition price. Unfortunately, he could not begin to afford even that discounted price.

We next used Strategy 5, "Consider Other Medications in the Same Class." Instead of prescribing the brand-name medicines, Prinivil®, Toprol-XL®, and Zocor®, I prescribed similar generic drugs in each of the brand-name drug class. Specifically, I prescribed lisinopril, instead of brand-name Altace® (both are ACE inhibitors), generic atenolol instead of brand-name Toprol-XL® (both are beta-blockers), and generic lovastatin instead of brand-name Zocor® (both are statins).

Jack then used Strategy 3, "Buy Generic Medicines." Through the Express Scripts Rx Outreach program he bought his generic drugs, lisinopril, atenolol, and lovastatin. Each generic medication cost him about a dollar a week through this program. Because he received a coated stent during his angioplasty, he requires Plavix®, for which there is no acceptable substitute. Jack could not afford the $100-plus monthly expense for this drug, and if he does not take it his coronary artery may clog up, causing a heart attack.

Using Strategy 7, "Use Pharmaceutical Assistance Programs," Jack enrolled in the Bristol-Myers Squibb Program for Plavix®. He received his medication within two weeks of submitting his form, and this program may save Jack from suffering a heart attack.

Pharmaceutical Assistance Programs

Jack is one of the millions of Americans who receive medications for free or at a substantial discount through a pharmaceutical assistance program. Each year, pharmaceutical companies donate billions of dollars of medications worldwide, and these companies are an excellent source of discounted or free medications. Many physicians' offices are well stocked with samples, and physicians frequently provide patients with medications for free. In some cases, pharmaceutical representatives have kept needy patients of mine continuously supplied with samples.

Patients, acting with their physicians, can apply to a large number of pharmaceutical programs that provide medications at a reduced cost or no cost. Dozens of pharmaceutical companies have pharmaceutical assistance programs to help the needy. The programs vary from manufacturer to manufacturer in the scope of products offered, patient or family income limits, and physicians' involvement. The duration of the programs varies as well; it is not clear if all of the programs will continue after 2006, when Medicare Part D goes into effect. There are several major websites to help access these programs.

In 1997, Libby Overly, M.Ed., MSW, was a social worker who had made a database about the prescription drug programs that she learned about to assist her patients. Dr. Richard Sagall was a family physician interested in developing a web-based project to help patients. They collaborated and launched the NeedyMeds website at www.needymeds.com. The site has expanded to include information on more than 250 programs and nearly 2,000 drugs and dosages. Many of the necessary drug companies' application forms are available on the site for downloading. Free information about discount prescription card programs, Medicaid programs, and other state programs is also provided. You don't need to provide any personal information to fully use the NeedyMeds website.

The Pharmaceutical Research and Manufacturers of America (PhRMA) have created websites, www.rxhope.com/pap_info.asp and www.helpingpatients.org/, where patients and physicians can search for medications by brand name or by pharmaceutical company. Searching the programs is free, and you do not need to register. Applications for some of the programs may be downloaded from the website. Other companies require a physician to request the application form. You may also request a Directory of Prescription Drug Patient Assistance Programs, which is sent free of charge, by telephoning 800-762-4636. Program information, including eligibility and contact information, has primarily been taken from the PhRMA websites for the following companies and drugs.

The newest website is the creation of the Partnership for Prescription Assistance, which brings together American drug companies and others, including the American Academy of Family Physicians, the NAACP, and the National Alliance for Hispanic Health, and the National Medical Association. It aims to offer "a single point of access to more than 275 public and private patient assistance programs, including more than 150 programs offered by pharmaceutical companies." The website, www.pparx.org, has sections dedicated to patients, caregivers, and doctors. Its toll-free phone number is 888-477-2669. This website has information that is similar to the RxHope and HelpingPatients websites.

Assistance is also available from other non-profit organizations. RxAssist is a national program supported by the Robert Wood Johnson

Foundation that has lists private organizations on its website at www.rxassist.org/. For example, Health Kentucky, a private, nonprofit organization that provides health care and pharmaceuticals for Kentucky residents, is listed on the RxAssist website. Health Kentucky's website is www.healthkentucky.org/what.html. The Needy Meds website, www.needymeds.com, also has listings for state and local programs.

SPECIFIC PROGRAMS

Merck, the manufacturer of many best-selling medications, such as Zocor®, and Cozaar®, does not require proof of income to participate in its pharmaceutical assistance program. The Merck program has a one-page form to be completed by the patient and doctor, signed by the physician, and then mailed to Merck. If you are accepted into the patient assistance program, Merck will provide up to a one-year supply of medications, to be mailed to the patient's home or the physician's office. This is a very straightforward program, and my patients have received thousands of doses of medicine from this program.

Other companies, such as Novartis and Pfizer, require financial documentation, including income tax returns. The GlaxoSmithKline program involves the continuing help of an advocate, generally a nurse or physician, to enroll patients.

DRUG DISCOUNT CARDS

Drug discount cards offer patients a discount off "retail" price at the point of service. Some patients and pharmacists have told me that the cards frequently provide little or no saving compared to finding the lowest price at a discount pharmacy.

The Together Rx™ program was developed in 2002 by a consortium of pharmaceutical companies, including Abbott Laboratories, AstraZeneca, Aventis, Bristol-Myers Squibb, GlaxoSmithKline, Janssen, Novartis, and Ortho-McNeil, to help income-eligible Medicare recipients. Individuals with annual incomes less than $28,000 or couples with annual incomes less than $38,000 are eligible, and more than 150 drugs are covered by the program. The average discount is estimated at 20 to 40 percent of retail prices. More information is available on the web at www.togetherrx.com. The website reports that the Together Rx card has saved 1.4 million cardholders and patients $640 million; however, my patients have reported modest savings when using such drug cards as compared with other programs and techniques.

Ten pharmaceutical companies, Abbott Laboratories, AstraZeneca, Bristol-Myers Squibb, GlaxoSmithKline, Jansseen, Novartis, Ortho-McNeil, Pfizer, Sanofi-Aventis, and Takeda, created a similar program. The Together Rx Access™ Program was created in January 2005 to provide discounted pharmaceuticals for certain individuals and families. The drug discount card program is available to legal U.S. residents under age 65 lacking prescription drug insurance, Medicare, or Medicaid with household income not exceeding the following: $30,000 for a single person, $40,000 for a couple, $50,000 for a family of three, $60,000 for a family of four, and $70,000 for a family of five. Those with a family of six and greater can contact Together Rx Access™ at 800-444-4106 to determine eligibility. The estimated savings on over 275 brand-name products is 25% to 40%. You can enroll in the program and see a listing of available medications at www.togetherrxaccess.com/.

In the following list, detailed information about the pharmaceutical assistance programs of the largest drug companies is followed by a table of more than 500 of the most prescribed medications in the United States. Both the generic and brand names are listed. Remember that these programs may be changed at any time. If you take a medication that is not on the list, your pharmacist can tell you the manufacturer of your medications, and you can use the following list to find the appropriate telephone number, when available, to get more information.

ABBOTT LABORATORIES PATIENT ASSISTANCE PROGRAM

The Abbott Laboratories Patient Assistance Program provides temporary assistance to low-income individuals who do not have, or do not qualify for prescription medication benefits through private insurance or government-funded programs such as Medicaid. The Abbott Laboratories Patient Assistance Program may be contacted by mail or telephone. Patient eligibility is determined by Abbott after the application is completed.

Abbott Laboratories Patient Assistance Program
Pharmaceutical Products Division
Dept. D-31C, J23
200 Abbott Park Road
Abbott Park, IL 60064-6161
Phone: 800-222-6885
Fax: 847-937-9826

SELECTED ABBOTT LABORATORIES MEDICATIONS AVAILABLE
Biaxin® (clarithromycin)
Depakote® (divalproex)
Gengraf® (cyclosporine)
HUMIRA® (adalimumab)
Kaletra® (lopinavir/ritonavir)
Mavik® (trandolapril)
Norvir® (ritonavir)
Synthroid® (levothyroxine)
Tarka® (trandolapril/verapamil)
TriCor® (fenofibrate)

You should telephone 800-448-6472 to inquire about HUMIRA® (adalimumab), as this drug is provided by a separate Abbott Laboratories Program. Kaletra® (lopinavir/ritonavir) and Norvir® (ritonavir) are provided by Abbott Virology™; applications are available by telephoning 800-222-6885 or on the Internet at www.AbbottVirology.com.

ASTRAZENECA FOUNDATION PATIENT ASSISTANCE PROGRAM
The AstraZeneca Foundation Patient Assistance Program provides assistance to low-income individuals who do not have or do not qualify for prescription medication benefits through private insurance or government-funded programs. According to the NeedyMeds website, patients must have an annual income below $18,000 per individual or $24,000 per couple to quality. The AstraZeneca Foundation Patient Assistance Program may be contacted by mail or telephone.

AstraZeneca Foundation Patient Assistance Program
P.O. Box 66651
St. Louis, MO 63166-6551
Phone: 800-424-3727

SELECTED ASTRAZENECA MEDICATIONS AVAILABLE
Accolate® (zafirlukast)
Arimidex® (anastrozole)
Atacand® (candesartan)
Casodex® (bicalutamide)
Crestor® (rosuvastatin)
Faslodex® (fulvestrant)
Nexium® (esomeprazole)
Nolvadex® (tamoxifen)
Plendil® (felodipine)
Pulmicort ® (budesonide)
Rhinocort Aqua® (budesonide)
Seroquel® (quetiapine)
Toprol-XL® (metoprolol succinate)
Zoladex® (goserelin acetate implant)

AVENTIS PATIENT ASSISTANCE PROGRAM
The Aventis Patient Assistance Program provides assistance to low-income U.S. residents who do not have or do not qualify for prescription medication benefits through private insurance or government-funded programs. According to the NeedyMeds website, the patient's total annual income must be at or below the following: $18,620 for an individual; $24,980 for a family of two; $31,340 for a family of three. The Aventis Patient Assistance Program may be contacted by mail or telephone.

Aventis Patient Assistance Program
P.O. Box 759
Somerville, NJ 08876
Phone: 800-221-4025

SELECTED AVENTIS MEDICATIONS AVAILABLE

Allegra® (fexofenadine)

Allegra D® (fexofenadine HCL and pseudoephedrine HCL)

Amaryl® (glimepiride)

Lantus® (insulin glargine)

Lovenox® (enoxaparin)Nasacort® AQ (triamcinolone acetonide)

Nilandron® (nilutamide)

You should telephone 888-632-8607 to inquire about Lovenox® (enoxaparin) or telephone 800-996-6626 to inquire about Nilandron® (nilutamide) as these drugs are covered by separate Aventis Programs.

BOEHRINGER INGELHEIM CARE FOUNDATION PATIENT ASSISTANCE PROGRAM

The Boehringer Ingelheim Care Foundation Patient Assistance Program makes most Boehringer Ingelheim products available to applicants who are without pharmaceutical insurance coverage and whose income is less than 200 percent of the Federal Poverty Guidelines. For an individual, 200 percent of the Federal Poverty Guidelines is $18,620, and for a couple, the amount is $24,980. This program is available to people of all ages, although an application can be sent only to those age 18 and older. To meet eligibility requirements, applicants must be U.S. citizens or legal residents who meet the financial and income criteria specified by the Boehringer Ingelheim Care Foundation. Applicants also must not qualify for prescription medication benefits through private insurance or government-funded programs. The Boehringer Ingelheim Care Foundation Patient Assistance Program may be contacted by mail or telephone.

Boehringer Ingelheim Care Foundation Patient Assistance Program

c/o Express Scripts Specialty Distribution Services, Inc.

P.O. Box 66555

St. Louis, MO 63166-6555

Phone: 800-556-8317

SELECTED BOEHRINGER INGELHEIM MEDICATIONS AVAILABLE
Aggrenox® (dipyridamole/aspirin)
Atrovent® (ipratropium) inhalation aerosol
Catapres-TTS® (clonidine hydrochloride)
Combivent® (ipratropium bromide/albuterol sulfate aerosol)
Flomax® (tamsulosin)
Micardis® (telmisartan)
Mobic® (meloxicam)
Spiriva® (tiotropium)
Viramune® (nevirapine)

BRISTOL-MYERS SQUIBB PATIENT ASSISTANCE FOUNDATION

The Bristol-Myers Squibb Patient Assistance Program provides assistance to applicants with a financial hardship who do not have, or do not qualify for, prescription medication benefits through private insurance or government-funded programs. Patient eligibility is determined by Bristol-Myers Squibb on a case-by-case basis. The Bristol-Myers Squibb Patient Assistance Foundation may be contacted by mail or telephone.

Bristol-Myers Squibb Patient Assistance Foundation
P.O. Box 1058
Somerville, NJ 08876
Phone: 800-736-0003, ext. 2

SELECTED BRISTOL-MYERS SQUIBB MEDICATIONS AVAILABLE
Avalide® (irbesartan/HCTZ)
Avapro® (irbesartan)
BuSpar® (buspirone)
Cefzil® (cefprozil)
Coumadin® (warfarin)
Desyrel® (trazodone)
Glucophage® (metformin)
Glucovance® (glyburide/metformin)
Kenalog® (nystatin/triamcinolone acetonide)
Monopril® (fosinopril)
Plavix® (clopidogrel)

Pravachol® (pravastatin)
Prolixin® (fluphenazine)
Pronestyl® (procainamide)
Sinemet® (carbidopa/levodopa)
Tequin® (gatifloxacin)

GLAXOSMITHKLINE PATIENT ASSISTANCE FOUNDATION

GlaxoSmithKline has three major patient assistance programs. They are Commitment to Access for cancer patients, Bridges to Access for indigent patients, and Orange Card^{SM} for Medicare recipients. Unlike many other pharmaceutical assistance programs, patients cannot directly access the Commitment to Access or the Bridges to Access. These programs involve the continuing help of a patient advocate to enroll patients. An advocate may be a physician, nurse, or social worker but cannot be a friend or family member of the patient. The advocate helps fills out the enrollment form and follows up with the applicant. Bridges to Access covers all GlaxoSmithKline outpatient medications.

GLAXOSMITHKLINE COMMITMENT TO ACCESS

The GlaxoSmithKline Commitment to Access program provides cancer drugs for patients who cannot afford them. To qualify, the applicant must be a resident of the United States with a household income of not more than 350 percent of the Federal Poverty Guidelines ($32,585 for a single person and $43,715 for a couple). The applicant must not be eligible for prescription drug benefits. An advocate may download an enrollment form from the GSK website at www.commitmenttoaccess.gsk.com. Alternatively, an advocate may contact the program by mail or telephone.

GlaxoSmithKline Commitment to Access
P.O. Box 29038
Phoenix, AZ 85038-9038
Phone: 866-265-6491

SELECTED GLAXOSMITHKLINE COMMITMENT TO ACCESS MEDICATIONS AVAILABLE
Hycamtin® (topotecan)
Leukeran® (chlorambucil)
Myleran® (busulfan)
Navelbine® (vinorelbine)
Tabloid® (thioguanine)
Zofran® (ondansetron)

GLAXOSMITHKLINE BRIDGES TO ACCESS
GlaxoSmithKline Bridges to Access also requires the continuing help of a patient advocate to enroll patients. To qualify, the applicant must be a resident of the United States and must live in either a single-person household with an income of not more than $25,000 per year or a multiperson household with total incomes less than 250 percent of the Federal Poverty Guidelines ($31,225 for a couple). The applicant must not be eligible for prescription drug benefits through any private or public insurer payer program. There is a $5 copayment for each refill of each medication. Program application forms are available from the Internet at www.bridgestobccess.gsk.com.

For all medications except cancer medications, the advocate should call 866-PATIENT (866-728-4368), Monday to Friday from 8:00 A.M. to 8:00 P.M. after an application form has been obtained and completed. For cancer medications, the advocate calls 866-265-6491. If the applicant is deemed eligible, then an identification number on the enrollment form is activated. The applicant can take the coupon with a prescription to any retail pharmacy to receive up to a sixty-day supply of the prescribed medicine for a $5 or $10 copayment per drug per fill. The representative will direct the advocate and applicant on mailing the application and supporting documentation.

Bridges to Access
P.O. Box 29038
Phoenix, AZ 85038-9038
Phone: 866-728-4368

GLAXOSMITHKLINE'S ORANGE CARD^{SM}

The GlaxoSmithKline Orange Card^{SM} program assists Medicare recipients. The applicant must be enrolled in Medicare with an annual income level at or below $30,000 for a single person or $40,000 for a couple. One may not be enrolled in any program that pays for prescription medications, such as a private secondary insurance, employer plan, Medigap, Medicare HMO, Medicaid, or state assistance program. Unlike the other GlaxoSmithKline programs, the patient may access the program directly, without the help of an advocate.

The Orange Card^{SM} should be shown to the pharmacist when buying the medications. Participants with an Orange Card^{SM} should save approximately 30 percent. You can apply for an Orange Card^{SM} by telephone or mail.

Orange Card^{SM} Program
P.O. Box 7812
Ocala, FL 34478-9805
Phone: 888-ORANGE6

SELECTED GLAXOSMITHKLINE MEDICATIONS AVAILABLE FOR ORANGE CARD^{SM} DISCOUNT AND BRIDGES TO ACCESS
Advair™ Diskus® (salmeterol/fluticasone)
Albenza® (albendazole)
Amerge® (naratriptan)
Amoxil® (amoxicillin)
Augmentin® (amoxicillin/clavulanate)
Avandia® (rosiglitazone)
Avodart™ (dutasteride)
Beconase® (beclomethasone)
Ceftin® (cefuroxime)
Coreg® (carvedilol)
Daraprim® (pyrimethamine)
Dyazide® (triamterene/hydrochlorothiazide)
Epivir® (lamivudine)
Flonase® (fluticasone)
Flovent® (fluticasone)

Imitrex® (sumatriptan)
Lamictal® (lamotrigine)
Paxil® (paroxetine)
Relenza® (zanamavir)
Requip® (ropinirole)
Serevent® (salmeterol xinafoate)
Valtrex® (valacyclovir)
Wellbutrin SR® (bupropion)
Zofran® (ondansetron)
Zyban® (bupropion)

LILLY CARES™ PATIENT ASSISTANCE PROGRAM

Lilly provides assistance to U.S. residents without Medicare who do not have private or public prescription coverage through its Lilly Cares™ program. Eligibility is based on the lack of prescription drug coverage, the patient's inability to pay, and is determined on a case-by-case basis.

Lilly Answers® is a separate program for Medicare patients lacking prescription drug insurance and with an income below $18,000 per individual or $24,000 per couple. Program information is available at www.lillyanswers.com or by calling 877-795-4559. Enrollees will receive a drug discount card and can purchase a 30-day supply of many Lilly drugs for $12/month at local pharmacies. Available drugs are listed in the following table. The Lilly Patient Assistance Program may be contacted by telephone or mail.

Lilly Cares™ Program Administrator
P.O. Box 230999
Centreville, VA 20120
Phone: 800-545-6962

SELECTED LILLY MEDICATIONS
Ceclor ® (cefaclor)
Cymbalta® (duloxetine)
Evista® (raloxifene)
Humalog® (Insulin Lispro Injection, [Recombinant DNA Orgin])

Humulin L® (Lente Human Insulin [Recombinant DNA Origin] Zinc Suspension)

Humulin N® (NPH Human Insulin [Recombinant DNA Origin] Isophane Suspension)

Humulin R® (Regular Insulin Human Injection, USP [Recombinant DNA Origin])

Humulin U® (Ultralente Human Insulin [Recombinant DNA Origin] Extended Zinc Suspension)

Prozac® (fluoxetine)

Zyprexa® (olanzapine)

MERCK PATIENT ASSISTANCE PROGRAM

The Merck patient assistance program provides free Merck medications to those eligible of all ages. You can qualify for the program if you meet the three following criteria: (1) Any U.S. resident with a prescription signed by a U.S. physician for a medication manufactured by Merck. You do not have to be an U.S. citizen; (2) No insurance or other coverage for prescription medications; (3) Annual income of $18,000 or less for an individual, $24,000 or less for a couple, or $35,000 or less for a family of four. The Merck Patient Assistance Program may be contacted by mail or telephone Monday through Friday from 8:00 A.M. to 8:00 P.M. An original application, not a photocopy, is required.

Merck Patient Assistance Program
P.O. Box 690
Horsham, PA 19044-9979
Phone: 800-727-5400

SELECTED MERCK MEDICATIONS AVAILABLE
Cozaar® (losartan)
Fosamax® (alendronate)
Hyzaar® (losartan/HCTZ)
Mevacor® (lovastatin)
Midamor® (amiloride)
Noroxin® (norfloxacin)
Proscar® (finasteride)

Singulair® (montelukast)
Timoptic® (timolol maleate ophthalmic solution)
Zocor® (simvastatin)

MERCK/SCHERING-PLOUGH PATIENT ASSISTANCE PROGRAM

Zetia™ (ezetimibe) and Vytorin™ (ezetimibe/simvastatin) are available through Merck/Schering-Plough patient assistance program, which has application criteria identical to those of the Merck program. If you qualify for the program, request an application by telephoning Merck/Schering-Plough for information about its patient assistance program at 800-347-7503 Monday through Friday from 8:00 A.M. to 8:00 P.M. An original application, not a photocopy, is required.

NOVARTIS PATIENT ASSISTANCE PROGRAM

Novartis provides assistance to U.S. residents who do not have private or public prescription coverage. Proof of income within program guidelines is required, including a copy of your most recent federal tax return. Patient eligibility is determined by Novartis after the application is completed. The Novartis Patient Assistance Program may be contacted by mail or telephone.

Novartis Patient Assistance Program
P.O. Box 66556
St. Louis, MO 63166-6556
Phone: 800-277-2254, option 3

SELECTED NOVARTIS MEDICATIONS AVAILABLE
Diovan® (valsartan)
Exelon® (rivastigmine)
Famvir® (famciclovir)
Lamisil® (terbinafine)
Lescol® (fluvastatin)
Lotrel® (amlodipine/benazepril)
Miacalcin® nasal spray (calcitonin-salmon nasal spray)
Ritalin LA® (methylphenidate hydrochloride)

Starlix® (nateglinide)
Tegretol® (carbamazepine)
Trileptal® (oxcarbazepine)
Zelnorm™ (tegaserod)

PFIZER CONNECTION TO CARE

To be eligible for the Pfizer Connection to Care program, you may not have any prescription drug coverage. This includes patients who have reached their caps under other plans, those in "generics only" plans, and those in any other insurance plans. The annual gross single household income must be $19,000 or less. The annual gross family household income must be $31,000 or less. To apply, applicants must submit an application, a copy of their prior year's tax return with supporting documentation, and an original signed prescription from their physician. Pfizer Connection to Care may be contacted by mail or telephone.

Pfizer Connection to Care
P.O. Box 66585
St. Louis, MO 63166-6585
Phone: 800-707-8990

SELECTED PFIZER MEDICATIONS AVAILABLE
Accupril® (quinapril)
Cardura® (doxazosin)
Diabinese® (chlorpropamide)
Glucotrol XL® (glipizide)
Lipitor® (atorvastatin)
Navane® (thiothixene)
Neurontin® (gabapentin)
Norvasc® (amlodipine)
Procardia® (nifedipine)
Procardia XL® (nifedipine)
Sinequan® (doxepin)
Viagra® (sildenafil citrate)
Zoloft® (sertraline)
Zyrtec® (cetirizine)

ROCHE LABS PATIENT ASSISTANCE PROGRAM

Roche Laboratories provides assistance to U.S. residents who do not have private or public prescription coverage and are unable to afford Roche products. Roche offers the Patient Assistance Program as a philanthropic endeavor to ensure access to Roche products for needy patients at no charge until alternative funding can be found. The Roche Labs Patient Assistance Program is not intended to supplant or replace prescription drug coverage provided by third-party public or private payers. Patient eligibility is determined on a case-by-case basis depending upon economic and insurance criteria. The Roche Labs Patient Assistance Program may be contacted by mail or telephone.

Roche Labs Patient Assistant Program
340 Kingsland Street
Nutley, NJ 07110-1100
Phone: 800-285-4484

SELECTED ROCHE LABORATORIES MEDICATIONS AVAILABLE
Accutane® (isotretinoin)
Anaprox® (naproxen)
Bumex® (bumetanide)
Cardene® (nicardipine)
Demadex® (torsemide)
Klonopin® (clonazepam)
Naprosyn® (naproxen)

Roche's drugs used to treat hepatitis C, Copegus® (ribavirin) and Pegasys® (peginterferon alfa-2a), are available through their Pegassist[SM] program that can be reached by telephoning 800-387-1258.

SCHERING LABORATORIES PATIENT ASSISTANCE PROGRAM

The Schering Laboratories Patient Assistance Program provides assistance to low-income U.S. residents who do not have, or do not qualify for, prescription medication benefits through private insurance or government-funded programs. Patient eligibility is determined on a case-by-case basis depending upon economic and insurance criteria. Eligibility criteria are subject to change at any time. The Schering

Laboratories Patient Assistance Program may be contacted by mail or telephone.

SP-Cares
Patient Assistance Program
P.O. Box 52122
Phoenix, AZ 85072
Phone: 800-656-9485

SELECTED SCHERING LABORATORIES MEDICATIONS AVAILABLE
Clarinex® (desloratadine)
Diprolene® AF cream (betamethasone dipropionate)
Imdur® (isosorbide mononitrate)
K-Dur® (potassium chloride)
Lotrisone® cream (clotrimazole/betamethasone)
Nasonex® (mometasone)
Nitro-Dur® patches (transdermal nitroglycerin)
Proventil® aerosol inhaler (albuterol aerosol inhaler)

Other Schering drugs, including Intron® A (interferon alfa-2b recombinant), Peg-Intron® (peginterferon alfa-2b), Rebetol® (ribavirin), and Temodar® (temozolomide) are available through its Commitment to Care™ Program. Eligibility is determined on a case by case basis. The Commitment to Care™ Program may be contacted by mail or telephone.

Commitment to Care™
1250 Bayhill Dr
Suite 300
San Bruno, CA 94066
Phone: 800-521-7157

WYETH PHARMACEUTICAL ASSISTANCE FOUNDATION
The Wyeth Pharmaceutical Assistance Foundation provides assistance to low-income U.S. residents who do not have, or do not qualify for, prescription medication benefits through private insurance or government-funded programs, and earn less than 200 percent of the

current Federal Poverty Guidelines ($18,620 for a single person and $24,980 for a couple). The Wyeth Pharmaceutical Assistance Foundation may be contacted by mail or telephone.

Wyeth Pharmaceutical Assistance Foundation
P.O. Box 1759
Paoli, PA 19301Phone: 800-568-9938

SELECTED WYETH MEDICATIONS AVAILABLE
Cordarone® (amiodarone)
Effexor XR® (venlafaxine)
Lodine® (etodolac)
Premarin® (conjugated estrogens)
Prempro™ (conjugated estrogens/medroxyprogesterone)
Protonix® (pantoprazole)

Medications and the Sponsoring Programs' Contact Numbers

BRAND NAME	GENERIC NAME	SPONSORING COMPANY	TELEPHONE
8-Mop	Methoxsalen	Valeant	800-556-1937, ext. 4
A/T/S®	Erythromycin gel	Medicis	800-550-5115
Abelcet®	Amphotericin B lipid complex injection	Enzon	800-345-2252
Abilify®	Aripiprazole	BMS	800-736-0003
Accolate®	Zafirlukast	AstraZeneca	800-424-3727
AccuNeb®	Albuterol	Dey	800-755-5560
Accupril®	Quinapril	Pfizer	800-717-6005
Accuretic®	Quinapril/HCTZ	Pfizer	800-717-6005
Accutane®	Isotretinoin	Roche	Not available
Aceon®	Perindopril	Solvay	800-256-8918
Aci-jel®	Therapeutic vaginal jelly	Ortho-McNeil	800-577-3788

Medications and the Sponsoring Programs' Contact Numbers cont.			
BRAND NAME	**GENERIC NAME**	**SPONSORING COMPANY**	**TELEPHONE**
Aciphex®	Rabeprazole	Janssen	800-523-5870
Aclovate®	Alclometasone dipropionate cream	GSK	866-728-4368
Acthrel®	Corticorelin ovine triflutate	Ferring	Not available
Actigall®	Ursodiol	Novartis	Not available
Actiq®	Fentanyl	Cephalon	877-229-1241
Activase®	Alteplase	Genentech	800-530-3083
Activella®	Estradiol/ norethindrone acetate	Novo Nordisk	866-668-6336
Actonel®	Risedronate	P&G	800-830-9049
Actos®	Pioglitazone	Takeda	800-830-9159
Adalat® CC	Nifedipine	Bayer	800-998-9180
Adderall XR®	Amphetamine sulfate, amphetamine aspartate, dextroamphetamine saccharate, dextroamphetamine sulfate	Shire	Not available
Advair™ Diskus®	Salmeterol/fluticasone	GSK	866-728-4368
Advicor®	Lovastatin/niacin	Kos	888-454-7437
AeroBid®	Flunisolide	Forest	800-851-0758
Agenerase®	Amprenavir	GSK	866-728-4368
Aggrastat®	Tirofiban	Merck	877-810-0595
Aggrenox®	Dipyridamole/aspirin	BI	800-556-8317
Agrylin®	Anagrelide	Shire	908-203-0657
Alavert™	Loratadine	Wyeth	800-568-9938

Medications and the Sponsoring Programs' Contact Numbers cont.

BRAND NAME	GENERIC NAME	SPONSORING COMPANY	TELEPHONE
Albenza®	Albendazole	GSK	866-728-4368
Aldactone®	Spironolactone	Pfizer	800-717-6005
Aldara™ cream	Imiquimod	3M	800 328-0255
Aldomet®	Methyldopa	Merck	Not available
Aldoril®	Methyldopa/HCTZ	Merck	800-727-5400
Aldurazyme®	Laronidase	Genzyme	800-745-4447, ext. 7808
Alesse®	Levonorgestrel/ ethinyl estradiol	Wyeth	Not available
Allegra®	Fexofenadine	Aventis	800-221-4025
Altace®	Ramipril	King	877-546-5332
Altocor®	Lovastatin	Andrx	Not available
Amaryl®	Glimepiride	Aventis	800-221-4025
Ambien®	Zolpidem	Sanofi	Not available
Amerge®	Naratriptan	GSK	866-728-4368
Amicar®	Aminocaproic acid	Xanodyne	877-926-6396
Amoxil®	Amoxicillin	GSK	866-728-4368
Anaplex® DM	Dextromethorphan/ brompheniramine	ECR	800-527-1955
Anaplex® HD	Phenylephrine/hydrocodone	ECR	800-527-1955
Anaprox®	Naproxen	Roche	877-757-6243
Ancobon®	Flucytosine	Valeant	800-556-1937, ext. 4
Androderm®	Testosterone transdermal system	Watson	800-385-4081

Medications and the Sponsoring Programs' Contact Numbers cont.

BRAND NAME	GENERIC NAME	SPONSORING COMPANY	TELEPHONE
Antabuse®	Disulfiram	Odyssey	Not available
Antivert®	Meclizine	Pfizer	800-717-6005
Anusol-HC®	Hydrocortisone cream	King	877-546-5332
Anzemet®	Dolasetron	Aventis	800-221-4025
Apresoline®	Hydralazine	Novartis	Not available
Apri®	Desogestrel/ethinyl estradiol	Barr	Not available
Aranesp®	Darbepoetin alfa	Amgen	800-272-9376
Arava®	Leflunomide	Aventis	800-221-4025
Aredia®	Pamidronate	Novartis	Not available
Aricept®	Donepezil	Pfizer	800-226-2072
Arimidex®	Anastrozole	AstraZeneca	800-424-3727
Arixtra®	Fondaparinux	Sanofi	Not available
Armour® Thyroid	Thyroid desiccated	Forest	800-851-0758
Arthrotec®	Diclofenac/misoprostol	Pfizer	800-717-1761
Asacol®	Mesalamine	P&G	800-830-9049
Aspirin	Aspirin	Bayer	Not available
Atacand HCT®	Candesartan/HCTZ	AstraZeneca	800-424-3727
Atacand®	Candesartan	AstraZeneca	800-424-3727
Atarax®	Hydroxyzine	Pfizer	Not available
Ativan®	Lorazepam	Wyeth	800-568-9938
Atrovent®	Ipratropium	BI	800-556-8317
Augmentin®	Amoxicillin/clavulanate	GSK	866-728-4368

Medications and the Sponsoring Programs' Contact Numbers cont.

BRAND NAME	GENERIC NAME	SPONSORING COMPANY	TELEPHONE
Avage™	Tazarotene	Allergan	Not available
Avalide®	Irbesartan/HCTZ	BMS	800-736-0003
Avandamet™	Rosiglitazone/metformin	GSK	866-728-4368
Avandia®	Rosiglitazone	GSK	866-728-4368
Avapro®	Irbesartan	BMS	800-736-0003
Avelox®	Moxifloxacin	Bayer	800-998-9180
Aviane®	Levonorgestrel/ ethinyl estradiol	Barr	Not available
Avodart®	Dutasteride	GSK	866-728-4368
Avonex®	Interferon beta-1a	Biogen	800-456-2255
Axert®	Almotriptan	Pfizer	800-717-6005
Axid®	Nizatidine	Lilly	Not available
Azmacort®	Triamcinolone acetonide	Aventis	800-221-4025
Azopt™	Brinzolamide	Alcon	800-222-8103, ext. 1
Azulfidine®	Sulfasalazine	Pfizer	800-707-8990
Bactrim®	Trimethoprim/ sulfamethoxazole	Roche	Not available
Bactroban® cream	Mupirocin calcium cream	GSK	866-728-4368
Beconase®	Beclomethasone dipropionate	GSK	866-728-4368
Benadryl®	Diphenhydramine	Pfizer	Not available
BeneFix®	Coagulation factor IX	Wyeth	888-999-2349
Benicar HCT™	Olmesartan	Sankyo	866-268-7327
Benicar™	Olmesartan	Sankyo	866-268-7327

Medications and the Sponsoring Programs' Contact Numbers cont.

BRAND NAME	GENERIC NAME	SPONSORING COMPANY	TELEPHONE
Bentyl®	Dicyclomine	Aventis	Not available
BenzaClin®	Clindamycin/benzoyl peroxide gel	Dermik	866-268-7326
Benzagel®	Benzoyl peroxide gel	Dermik	866-268-7326
Benzamycin®	Erythromycin/benzoyl peroxide gel	Dermik	866-268-7326
Betagan®	Levobunolol	Allergan	800-553-6783
Betapace AF®	Sotalol	Berlex	888-237-5394
Betaseron®	Interferon beta-1b	Berlex	800-948-5777
Betoptic S®	Betaxolol	Alcon	800-222-8103, ext. 1
Bextra®	Valdecoxib	Pfizer	800-717-6005
Biaxin®	Clarithromycin	Abbott	800-865-7211
BiCitra®	Sodium citrate/ citric acid oral solution	Ortho-McNeil	800-577-3788
BiCNU®	Carmustine	BMS	800-272-4878
Blenoxane®	Bleomycin	BMS	800-272-4878
Blocadren®	Timolol	Merck	Not available
Bumex®	Bumetanide	Roche	Not available
Bupap®	Butalbital/acetaminophen	ECR	800-527-1955
Buphenyl®	Phenylbutyrate	Medicis	800-711-0811
BuSpar®	Buspirone	BMS	800-736-0003
Caduet®	Amlodipine/atorvastatin	Pfizer	800-707-8990
Calan®	Verapamil	Pfizer	Not available

Medications and the Sponsoring Programs' Contact Numbers cont.

BRAND NAME	GENERIC NAME	SPONSORING COMPANY	TELEPHONE
CamPath®	Alemtuzumab	Berlex	800-473-5832
Camptosar®	Irinotecan	Pfizer	877-744-5473
Capoten®	Captopril	Apothecon	Not available
Capozide®	Captopril/HCTZ	Apothecon	Not available
Carac™	Fluorouracil cream	Dermik	866-268-7326
Carafate®	Sucralfate	Aventis	800-221-4025
Cardene®	Nicardipine	Roche	800-285-4484
Cardizem CD®	Diltiazem	Biovail	866-268-7325
Cardura®	Doxazosin	Pfizer	800-707-8990
Cartia XT™	Diltiazem	Andrx	Not available
Casodex®	Bicalutamide	AstraZeneca	800-424-3727
Catapres-TTS®	Clonidine	BI	800-556-8317
Ceclor®	Cefaclor	Lilly	800-545-6962
CeeNU®	Lomustine	BMS	800-272-4878
Ceftin®	Cefuroxime	GSK	866-726-4368
Cefzil®	Cefprozil	BMS	800-736-0003
Celebrex®	Celecoxib	Pfizer	800-717-6005
Celexa®	Citalopram	Forest	800-851-0758
Celontin®	Methsuximide	Pfizer	Not available
Cenestin®	Synthetic conjugated estrogen	Duramed	800-425-3122
Ceredase®	Alglucerase	Genzyme	800-745-4447, ext. 7808

Medications and the Sponsoring Programs' Contact Numbers cont.

BRAND NAME	GENERIC NAME	SPONSORING COMPANY	TELEPHONE
Cerezyme®	Imiglucerase	Genzyme	800-745-4447, ext. 7808
Cialis®	Tadalafil	Lilly	Not available
Cinobac®	Cinoxacin	Oclassen	800-288-4508
Cipro®	Ciprofloxacin	Bayer	800-998-9180
Claforan®	Cefotaxime	Aventis	Not available
Clarinex®	Desloratadine	Schering	800-656-9485
Claritin®	Loratadine	Schering	Not available
Cleocin®	Clindamycin	Pfizer	800-717-6005
Climara®	Estrogen patch	Berlex	888-237-5394
Clinoril®	Sulindac	Merck	Not available
Clorpres®	Clonidine/chlorthalidone	Bertek	888-823-7835
Clozapine®	Clozapine	Ivax	800-507-8334
Clozaril®	Clozapine	Novartis	800-277-2254
Cognex®	Tacrine	First Horizon	800-869-4514
Combivent®	Ipratropium/ albuterol inhaler	BI	800-556-8317
Combivir®	Lamivudine/zidovudine	GSK	866-726-4368
Compazine®	Prochlorperazine	GSK	866-728-4368
Concerta®	Methylphenidate	McNeil	866-727-4626
Condylox®	Podofilox gel	Oclassen	800-288-4508
Copegus®	Ribavirin	Roche	800-387-1258
Cordarone®	Amiodarone	Wyeth	800-568-9938

Medications and the Sponsoring Programs' Contact Numbers cont.

BRAND NAME	GENERIC NAME	SPONSORING COMPANY	TELEPHONE
Cordran®	Flurandrenolide lotion	Oclassen	800-288-4508
Coreg®	Carvedilol	GSK	866-728-4368
Corgard®	Nadolol	King	877-546-5332
Cormax™	Clobetasol propionate cream	Oclassen	800-288-4508
Cosmegen®	Dactinomycin	Merck	800-727-5400
Cosopt®	Dorzolamide/ timolol maleate	Merck	800-994-2111
Cotrim®	Trimethoprim/ sulfamethoxazole	Teva	Not available
Coumadin®	Warfarin	BMS	800-736-0003
Covera-HS®	Verapamil	Pfizer	800-717-6005
Cozaar®	Losartan	Merck	800-727-5400
Crestor®	Rosuvastatin	AstraZeneca	800-424-3727
Crixivan®	Indinavir	Merck	800-850-3430
Cuprimine®	Penicillamine	Merck	800-727-5400
Curosurf®	Poractant alfa	Dey	800-755-5560
Cymbalta®	Duloxetine	Lilly	800-545-6962
Cystadane®	Betaine anhydrous solution	Orphan	800-999-6673
CytoGam®	Cytomegalovirus immune globulin	MedImmune	Not available
Cytomel®	Liothyronine	Jones	877-757-6243
Cytoxan®	Cyclophosphamide	BMS	800-272-4878
D.H.E. 45®	Dihydroergotamine injection	Xcel	800-511-2120
Daraprim®	Pyrimethamine	GSK	866-728-4368

Medications and the Sponsoring Programs' Contact Numbers cont.			
BRAND NAME	**GENERIC NAME**	**SPONSORING COMPANY**	**TELEPHONE**
Darvocet-N®	Propoxyphene/ acetaminophen	NeoSan	Not available
DaunoXome®	Daunorubicin citrate liposome injection	Gilead	800-226-2056
DDAVP®	Desmopressin	Aventis	800-221-4025
Decadron®	Dexamethasone	Merck	800-727-5400
Declomycin®	Demeclocycline	ESP Pharma	800-319-4031
Deltasone®	Prednisone	Pfizer	Not available
Demadex®	Torsemide	Roche	Not available
Demser®	Metyrosine	Merck	800-727-5400
Depakote®	Divalproex	Abbott	Not available
Depocyt®	Cytarabine liposome	Chiron	800-775-7533
Desogen®	Desogestrel/ethinyl estradiol	Organon	Not available
Desyrel®	Trazodone	BMS	800-736-0003
Detrol® LA	Tolterodine	Pfizer	800-717-6005
Dexedrine®	Dextroamphetamine	GSK	866-728-4368
Dexferrum®	Iron dextran injection	American Regent	800-282-7712
Diaßeta®	Glyburide	Aventis	800-221-4025
Diastat®	Diazepam rectal gel	Xcel	Not available
Diflucan®	Fluconazole	Pfizer	800-717-6005
Digitek®	Digoxin	Bertek	Not available
Dilacor XR®	Diltiazem	Watson	Not available
Dilantin®	Phenytoin	Pfizer	800-717-6005

Medications and the Sponsoring Programs' Contact Numbers cont.

BRAND NAME	GENERIC NAME	SPONSORING COMPANY	TELEPHONE
Diovan HCT®	Valsartan/HCTZ	Novartis	800-277-2254
Diovan®	Valsartan	Novartis	800-277-2254
Dipentum®	Olsalazine	Celltech	866-523-3994
Ditropan XL®	Oxybutynin	Ortho-McNeil	800-577-3788
Diuril®	Chlorothiazide	Merck	800-727-5400
Dolobid®	Diflunisal	Merck	800-727-5400
Dostinex®	Cabergoline	Pfizer	800-717-1761
Dovonex®	Calcipotriene	BMS	800-736-0003
Doxil®	Doxorubicin liposome injection	Ortho Biotech	800-609-1083
Droxia®	Hydroxyurea	BMS	800-272-4878
DuoNeb™	Ipratropium/ albuterol inhaler	Dey	800-755-5560
Duragesic®	Fentanyl transdermal system	Janssen	800-652-6227
Dyazide®	Triamterene/HCTZ	GSK	866-728-4368
Dynacin®	Minocycline	Medicis	800-711-0811
DynaCirc-CR®	Isradipine	Reliant	866-792-2737
Dynapen®	Dicloxacillin	BMS	800-736-0003
Effexor XR®	Venlafaxine	Wyeth	800-568-9938
Efudex®	Fluorouracil cream	Valeant	800-556-1937, ext. 4
Elavil®	Amitriptyline	AstraZeneca	Not available
Elmiron®	Pentosan polysulfate sodium	Ortho-McNeil	800-577-3788

Medications and the Sponsoring Programs' Contact Numbers cont.

BRAND NAME	GENERIC NAME	SPONSORING COMPANY	TELEPHONE
Enbrel®	Etanercept	Amgen	888-436-2735
Endocet®	Acetaminophen/oxycodone	Endo	Not available
Entocort™ EC	Budesonide	AstraZeneca	800-424-3727
EpiPen®	Epinephrine	Dey	800-755-5560
Epivir®	Lamivudine	GSK	866-728-4368
Epogen®	Epoetin alfa	Amgen	800-508-8090
Erbitux®	Cetuximab	ImClone	Not available
Esgic®	Butalbital/acetaminophen/ caffeine	Forest	Not available
Eskalith CR®	Lithium	GSK	888-672-6436
Estrace®	Estradiol	Warner Chilcott	Not available
Estring®	Estradiol	Pfizer	800-717-1761
Ethyol®	Amifostine	MedImmune	800-887-2467
Etopophos®	Etoposide	BMS	800-272-4878
Eulexin®	Flutamide	Schering	800-521-7157
Evista®	Raloxifene	Lilly	800-545-6962
Fabrazyme®	Agalsidase beta	Genzyme	800-745-4447 ext. 7808
Famvir®	Famciclovir	Novartis	800-277-2254
Faslodex®	Fulvestrant	AstraZeneca	800-424-3727
Felbatol®	Felbamate	Medpointe	800-678-4657
Femara®	Letrozole	Novartis	800-282-7630, ext. 2, then 2

Medications and the Sponsoring Programs' Contact Numbers cont.

BRAND NAME	GENERIC NAME	SPONSORING COMPANY	TELEPHONE
Ferrlecit®	Sodium ferric gluconate injection	Watson	888-964-4766, ext. 3
Flagyl®	Metronidazole	Pfizer	800-717-6005
Flexeril®	Cyclobenzaprine	Alza	800-865-7211
Flomax®	Tamsulosin	BI	800-556-8317
Flonase®	Fluticasone	GSK	866-728-4368
Florinef®	Fludrocortisone	King	877-546-5332
Flovent®	Fluticasone	GSK	866-728-4368
Floxin®	Ofloxacin	Ortho-McNeil	800-577-3788
Fludara®	Fludarabine	Berlex	800-473-5832
Focalin®	Dexmethylphenidate	Novartis	800-277-2254, ext. 2
Foradil®	Formoterol	Novartis	800-277-2254, ext. 2
Fortaz®	Ceftazidime	GSK	66-728-4368
Fosamax®	Alendronate	Merck	800-727-5400
Fototar®	Coal tar	Valeant	800-556-1937, ext. 4
Fragmin®	Delteparin	Pfizer	Not available
Gabitril®	Tiagabine	Cephalon	877-229-1241
Galzin™	Zinc acetate	Gate	800-292-4283, ext 3405
Gammagard® S/D	Immunoglobulin G	Baxter	800-888-4502
Gastrocrom®	Cromolyn	Celltech	866-523-3994
Gemzar®	Gemcitabine	Lilly	Not available
Genotropin®	Somatropin (Recombinant DNA Origin)	Pfizer	800-645-1280

Medications and the Sponsoring Programs' Contact Numbers cont.

BRAND NAME	GENERIC NAME	SPONSORING COMPANY	TELEPHONE
Geocillin®	Carbenicillin	Pfizer	Not available
Geodon®	Ziprasidone	Pfizer	800-717-6005
Gleevec®	Imatinib	Novartis	800-282-7630, ext. 2, then 2
Glucophage® XR	Metformin	BMS	800-736-0003
Glucotrol XL®	Glipizide	Pfizer	800-717-6005
Glucotrol®	Glipizide	Pfizer	800-717-6005
Glucovance®	Metformin/glyburide	BMS	800-736-0003
Glyset®	Miglitol	Pfizer	800-717-1761
Grifulvin V®	Griseofulvin	Ortho-McNeil	800-577-3788
Haldol®	Haloperidol	Ortho-McNeil	800-577-3788
Hectorol®	Doxercalciferol	Bone Care International	888-389-4242
Hepsera®	Adefovir	Gilead	800-226-2056
Herceptin®	Trastuzumab	Genentech	800-530-3083
Hexalen®	Altretamine	MGI	888-743-5711
Hiprex®	Methenamine	Aventis	800-221-4025
Humatrope®	Somatropin (Recombinant DNA Origin)	Lilly	800-847-6988
HUMIRA®	Adalimumab	Abbot	866-323-0661
Humulin®	Human insulin (Recombinant DNA Origin)	Lilly	800-545-6962
Hycamtin®	Topotecan	GSK	866-265-6491
Hydrea®	Hydroxyurea	BMS	800-272-4878
HydroDIURIL®	Hydrochlorothiazide	Merck	Not available
Hygroton®	Chlorthalidone	Aventis	Not available

Medications and the Sponsoring Programs' Contact Numbers cont.

BRAND NAME	GENERIC NAME	SPONSORING COMPANY	TELEPHONE
Hytone®	Hydrocortisone cream	Dermik	866-268-7326
Hytrin®	Terazosin	Abbott	Not available
Hyzaar®	Losartan/HCTZ	Merck	800-727-5400
Ifex®	Ifosfamide	BMS	800-272-4878
Imdur®	Isosorbide mononitrate	Schering/Key	800-656-9485
Imitrex®	Sumatriptan	GSK	866-728-4368
Inderal®	Propranolol	Wyeth	800-568-9938
Inderide®	Propranolol/HCTZ	Wyeth	800-568-9938
Indocin®	Indomethacin	Merck	Not available
INFeD®	Iron dextran	Watson	888-964-4766, ext. 3
InnoPran XL™	Propranolol	Reliant	Not available
Inspra™	Eplerone	Pfizer	800-717-6005
Intal®	Cromolyn	King	877-546-5332
Integrilin™	Eptifibatide	Millenium	800-232-8723
Intron A®	Interferon alfa-2b	Schering	800-521-7157
Inversine®	Mecamylamine	Merck	Not available
Ismo®	Isosorbide mononitrate	ESP Pharma	800-319-4031
Isoptin®	Verapamil	Abbott	Not available
Isopto Carpine®	Pilocarpine	Alcon	800-222-8103, ext. 1
Isordil®	Isosorbide dinitrate	Wyeth	Not available
Kaletra®	Lopinavir/ritonavir	Abbott	800-222-6885
K-Dur®	Potassium chloride	Schering/Key	800-656-9485
Keflex®	Cephalexin	Lilly	800-545-6962

Medications and the Sponsoring Programs' Contact Numbers cont.

BRAND NAME	GENERIC NAME	SPONSORING COMPANY	TELEPHONE
Kemadrin®	Procyclidine	King	877-546-5332
Kenalog®	Triamcinolone acetonide	BMS	800-736-0003
Kerlone®	Betaxolol	Sanofi	800-446-6267
Kineret™	Anakinra	Amgen	866-546-3738
Klaron®	Sulfacetamide lotion	Dermik	866-268-7326
Klonopin®	Clonazepam	Roche	800-285-4484
Klor-Con®	Potassium chloride	Upsher-Smith	800-654-2299
Klotrix®	Potassium chloride	BMS	800-736-0003
Lacrisert®	Hydroxypropyl cellulose ophthalmic insert	Merck	800-637-2568
Lamictal®	Lamotrigine	GSK	866-728-4368
Lamisil®	Terbinafine	Novartis	800-277-2254, ext. 2
Lamprene®	Clofazimine	Novartis	Not available
Lanoxicaps®	Digoxin	GSK	866-728-4368
Lanoxin®	Digoxin	GSK	866-728-4368
Lantus®	Insulin glargine (Recombinant DNA Origin)	Aventis	800-221-4025
Lasix®	Furosemide	Aventis	800-865-7211
Lescol®	Fluvastatin	Novartis	800-277-2254, ext. 2
Leukeran®	Chlorambucil	GSK	866-265-6491
Leukine®	Sargramostim	Berlex	800-473-5832
Leustatin®	Cladribine	Ortho Biotech	800-553-3851
Levaquin®	Levofloxacin	Ortho-McNeil	800-577-3788
Levitra®	Vardenafil	GSK	Not available

Medications and the Sponsoring Programs' Contact Numbers cont.

BRAND NAME	GENERIC NAME	SPONSORING COMPANY	TELEPHONE
Levothroid®	Levothyroxine	Forest	800-851-0758
Levoxyl®	Levothyroxine	King	877-546-5332
Lexapro®	Escitalopram	Forest	800-851-0758
Lidex®	Fluocinonide cream	Medicis	800-711-0811
Lidoderm®	Lidocaine	Endo	908-684-5799
Lipitor®	Atorvastatin	Pfizer	800-717-6005
Lodine®	Etodolac	Wyeth	800-568-9938
Lodosyn®	Carbidopa/levodopa	BMS	800-736-0003
Lodrane®	Brompheniramine/ pseudoephedrine	ECR	800-527-1955
Loestrin®	Norethindrone/ ethinyl estradiol	Pfizer	Not available
Lofibra®	Fenofibrate	Teva	Not available
Lopid®	Gemfibrozil	Pfizer	800-717-6005
Lopressor®	Metoprolol tartrate	Novartis	Not available
Loprox®	Ciclopirox solution	Medicis	800-711-0811
Lotensin HCT®	Benazepril/HCTZ	Novartis	800-277-2254, ext. 2
Lotensin®	Benazepril	Novartis	800-277-2254, ext. 2
Lotrel®	Amlodipine/benazepril	Novartis	800-277-2254, ext. 2
Lotrisone® cream	Clotrimazole/betamethasone	Schering	800-656-9485
Lotronex®	Alosteron	GSK	866-728-4368
Lovenox®	Enoxaparin	Aventis	888-632-8607
Lumigan®	Bimatoprost	Allergan	800-553-6783

Medications and the Sponsoring Programs' Contact Numbers cont.

BRAND NAME	GENERIC NAME	SPONSORING COMPANY	TELEPHONE
Lupron®	Leuprolide	Tap	800-830-1015
Lustra®	Hydroquinone cream	Medicis	800-550-5115
Lysodren®	Mitotane	BMS	800-272-4878
Macrobid®	Nitrofurantoin	P&G	800-830-9049
Malarone®	Atovaquone/proguanil	GSK	866-728-4368
Mandol®	Cefamandole	Lilly	800-545-6962
Materna®	Prenatal vitamins	Wyeth	Not available
Mavik®	Trandolapril	Abbott	800-222-6885
Maxair™	Pirbuterol	3M	800 328-0255
Maxalt®	Rizatriptan	Merck	800-727-5400
Maxzide®	Triamterene/HCTZ	Bertek	888-823-7835
Medrol®	Methylprednisolone	Pfizer	800-717-6005
Megace®	Megestrol	BMS	800-272-4878
Menest®	Esterified estrogen	King	877-546-5332
Mephyton®	Phytonadione	Merck	800-727-5400
Mepron®	Atovaquone	GSK	866-728-4368
Meridia®	Sibutramine	Abbott	Not available
Mesnex®	Mesna	BMS	800-272-4878
Mestinon®	Pyridostigmine	Valeant	800-556-1937, ext. 4
Metaglip™	Glipizide/metformin	BMS	800-865-7211
MetroCream®	Metronidazole cream	Galderma	800-582-8225
MetroGel- Vaginal®	Metronidazole	3M	800 328-0255

Medications and the Sponsoring Programs' Contact Numbers cont.

BRAND NAME	GENERIC NAME	SPONSORING COMPANY	TELEPHONE
MetroGel®	Metronidazole gel	Galderma	800-582-8225
MetroLotion®	Metronidazole lotion	Galderma	800-582-8225
Mevacor®	Lovastatin	Merck	800-727-5400
Miacalcin®	Calcitonin	Novartis	800-277-2254
Micardis HCT®	Telmisartan/HCTZ	BI	800-556-8317
Micardis®	Telmisartan	BI	800-556-8317
Microgestin®	Norethindrone/ ethinyl estradiol	Watson	Not available
Micro-K®	Potassium chloride	Whitehall-Robins	Not available
Micronase®	Glyburide	Pfizer	800-717-6005
Migranal®	Dihydroergotamine nasal spray	Xcel	800-511-2120
Minipress®	Prazosin	Pfizer	800-717-6005
Minitran™	Transdermal nitroglycerin patches	3M	800 328-0255
Minizide®	Prazosin/polythiazide	Pfizer	800-717-6005
Minocin®	Minocycline	Wyeth	800-568-9938
Mirapex®	Pramipexole	BI	800-556-8317
Mircette®	Desogestrel/ ethinyl estradiol	Organon	Not available
Moban®	Molindone	Endo	908-684-5799
Mobic®	Meloxicam	BI	800-556-8317
Modicon®	Norethindrone/ ethinyl estradiol	Ortho-McNeil	Not available

Medications and the Sponsoring Programs' Contact Numbers cont.

BRAND NAME	GENERIC NAME	SPONSORING COMPANY	TELEPHONE
Monistat-Derm®	Miconazole nitrate cream	Ortho-McNeil	800-577-3788
Monodox®	Doxycycline	Oclassen	800-288-4508
Monopril®	Fosinopril	BMS	800-736-0003
Monopril®-HCT	Fosinopril/HCTZ	BMS	800-736-0003
Motrin®	Ibuprofen	Ortho-McNeil	Not available
MS Contin®	Morphine	Purdue	800-599-6070
Mustargen®	Mechlorethamine	Merck	800-727-5400
Mutamycin®	Mitomycin C	BMS	800-272-4878
Mycelex®-G	Clotrimazole	Ortho-McNeil	800-577-3788
Mycobutin®	Rifabutin	Pfizer	800-717-1761
Mycolog® II cream	Triamcinolone acetonide/ nystatin	BMS	800-736-0003
Mycostatin®	Nystatin	BMS	800-736-0003
Myleran®	Busulfan	GSK	866-265-6491
Mylotarg™	Gemtuzumab	Wyeth	Not available
Mysoline®	Primidone	Xcel	Not available
Namenda™	Memantine	Forest	Not available
Naprosyn®	Naproxen	Roche	Not available
Nardil®	Phenelzine	Pfizer	Not available
Nasacort® AQ	Triamcinolone acetonide	Aventis	800-221-4025
Nasatab® LA	Guaifenesin/ pseudoephedrine	ECR	800-527-1955
Nasonex®	Mometasone furoate monohydrate	Schering	800-656-9485

Medications and the Sponsoring Programs' Contact Numbers cont.

BRAND NAME	GENERIC NAME	SPONSORING COMPANY	TELEPHONE
Naturetin®	Bendroflumethiazide	BMS	800-736-0003
Navane®	Thiothixene	Pfizer	800-717-6005
Navelbine®	Vinorelbine	GSK	866-265-6491
NebuPent®	Pentamidine aerosolized	American Pharmaceutical Partners	847-330-1289
Necon®	Norethindrone/ ethinyl estradiol	Watson	Not available
Neulasta®	Pegfilgrastim	Amgen	800-272-9376
Neumega®	Oprelvekin	Wyeth	888-638-6342
Neupogen®	Filgrastim	Amgen	800-272-9376
Neurontin®	Gabapentin	Pfizer	800-717-6005
Neutra-Phos®	Sodium phosphate/ potassium phosphate	Ortho-McNeil	800-577-3788
NeuTrexin®	Trimetrexate glucuronate	MedImmune	Not available
Nexium®	Esomeprazole	AstraZeneca	800-424-3727
Niacor®	Niacin	Upsher-Smith	800-654-2299
Niaspan®	Extended-release niacin	Kos	888-454-7437
Nilandron®	Nilutamide	Aventis	800-996-6626
Nitrek®	Transdermal nitroglycerin patches	Bertek	888-823-7835
Nitro-Dur® patches	Transdermal nitroglycerin patches	Schering	800-656-9485
Nitrolingual®	Nitroglycerin	First Horizon	800-869-4514
Nizoral®	Ketoconazole	Janssen	800-652-6227

Medications and the Sponsoring Programs' Contact Numbers cont.

BRAND NAME	GENERIC NAME	SPONSORING COMPANY	TELEPHONE
Nolvadex®	Tamoxifen	AstraZeneca	800-424-3727
Norflex™	Orphenadrine	3M	800 328-0255
Norgesic™	Orphenadrine/ aspirin/caffeine	3M	800 328-0255
Noritate®	Metronidazole cream	Dermik	866-268-7326
Noroxin®	Norfloxacin	Merck	800-727-5400
Norpace®	Disopyramide	Pfizer	800-717-6005
Norvasc®	Amlodipine	Pfizer	800-717-6005
Norvir®	Ritonavir	Abbott	800-222-6885
Novolin®	Human insulin isophane suspension (Recombinant DNA Origin)	Novo Nordisk	800-727-6500, ext. 3
Nutropin®	Somatropin (Recombinant DNA Origin)	Genentech	800-545-0498
Omnicef®	Cefdinir	Medicis	Not available
Ontak®	Denileukin diftitox	Ligand	877-654-4263
Orap®	Pimozide	Gate	800-292-4283, ext 3405
Ortho Tri-Cyclen®	Norgestimate/ ethinyl estradiol	Ortho-McNeil	Not available
Ortho-Cept®	Desogestrel/ethinyl estradiol	Ortho-McNeil	Not available
Ortho-Prefest™	Norgestimate/ ethinyl estradiol	King	877-546-5332
Oruvail®	Ketoprofen	Wyeth	800-568-9938
Ovide®	Malathion lotion	Medicis	800-550-5115
Oxistat®	Oxiconazole nitrate lotion	GSK	866-728-4368

Medications and the Sponsoring Programs' Contact Numbers cont.

BRAND NAME	GENERIC NAME	SPONSORING COMPANY	TELEPHONE
Oxsoralen®	Methoxsalen	Valeant	800-556-1937 ,ext. 4
Oxycontin®	Oxycodone	Purdue	800-599-6070
Pacerone®	Amiodarone	Upsher-Smith	800-654-2299
Pamelor®	Nortriptyline	Mallinckrodt	Not available
Pancrease®	Lipase/protease/amylase	Ortho-McNeil	800-482-1896
Panretin®	litretinoin gel	Ligand	877-654-4263
Parafon Forte®	Chlorzoxazone	Ortho-McNeil	800-482-1896
Paraplatin®	Carboplatin	BMS	800-272-4878
Parnate®	Tranylcypromine	GSK	866-728-4368
Paxil®	Paroxetine	GSK	866-728-4368
Pegasys®	Peginterferon alfa-2a	Roche	800-387-1258
Peg-intron®	Peginterferon alfa-2b	Schering	800-656-9485
Penlac™	Ciclopirox solution	Dermik	866-268-7326
Pentoxil®	Pentoxifylline	Upsher-Smith	800-654-2299
Pepcid®	Famotidine	Merck	800-727-5400
Percocet®	Acetaminophen/oxycodone	Endo	Not available
Phenergan®	Promethazine	Wyeth	Not available
Phenytek®	Phenytoin	Bertek	888-823-7835
Phospholine®	Echothiophate	Wyeth	800-568-9938
Phrenilin®	Butalbital/APAP	Amarin	866-262-7468
Platinol®-AQ	Cisplatin	BMS	800-272-4878
Plavix®	Clopidogrel	Sanofi	800-446-6267
Plendil®	Felodipine	AstraZeneca	800-424-3727

Medications and the Sponsoring Programs' Contact Numbers cont.

BRAND NAME	GENERIC NAME	SPONSORING COMPANY	TELEPHONE
Pletal®	Cilostazol	Otsuka	800-992-4546
Plexion®	Sodium sulfacetamide	Medicis	Not available
Pneumotussin®	Guaifenesin/hydrocodone	ECR	800-527-1955
Ponstel®	Mefenamic acid	First Horizon	800-869-4514
Prandin®	Repaglinide	Novo Nordisk	800-727-6500
Pravachol®	Pravastatin	BMS	800-736-0003
Pravigard™ PAC	Pravastatin/buffered aspirin	BMS	800-736-0003
Precose®	Acarbose	Bayer	800-998-9180
Prelone®	Prednisolone syrup	Muro	800-225-0974, ext. 3
Premarin®	Conjugated estrogens	Wyeth	800-568-9938
Premphase®	Conjugated estrogens/ medroxyprogesterone	Wyeth	800-568-9938
Prempro™	Conjugated estrogens/ medroxyprogesterone	Wyeth	800-568-9938
Prevacid®	Lansoprazole	Tap	800-830-1015
Prevalite®	Cholestyramine	Upsher-Smith	800-654-2299
Prinivil®	Lisinopril	Merck	800-727-5400
Prinzide®	Lisinopril/ hydrochlorothiazide	Merck	800-727-5400
Proamatine®	Midodrine	Shire	908-203-0657
Procanbid®	Procainamide	King	877-546-5332
Procardia®	Nifedipine	Pfizer	800-717-6005
Procrit®	Epoetin alfa	Ortho Biotech	800-553-3851
Proctocort®	Hydrocortisone	King	877-546-5332

Medications and the Sponsoring Programs' Contact Numbers cont.

BRAND NAME	GENERIC NAME	SPONSORING COMPANY	TELEPHONE
Proleukin®	Aldesleukin	Chiron	800-775-7533
Prolixin®	Fluphenazine	BMS	800-736-0003
Pronestyl®	Procainamide	BMS	800-736-0003
Proscar®	Finasteride	Merck	800-727-5400
Protonix®	Pantoprazole	Wyeth	800-568-9938
Protopic®	Tacrolimus ointment	Fujisawa	800-477-6472
Protropin®	Somatrem	Genentech	800-545-0498
Proventil®	Albuterol inhaler	Schering	800-656-9485
Provera®	Medroxyprogesterone	Pfizer	800-717-6005
Provigil®	Modafinil	Cephalon	877-229-1241
Prozac	Fluoxetine	Lilly	800-545-6962
Psorcon®	Diflorasone diacetate ointment	Dermik	866-268-7326
Pulmicort turbuhaler®	Budesonide inhalation powder	AstraZeneca	800-424-3727
Pulmozyme®	Dornase alfa inhalation solution	Genentech	800-297-5557
Purinethol®	Mercaptopurine	GSK	866-265-6491
Questran®	Cholestyramine	BMS	Not available
Quibron®-T	Theophylline	King	877-546-5332
Quibron®-T/SR	Theophylline/guaifenesin	King	877-546-5332
Quinidex®	Quinidine	Wyeth	Not available
Rapamune®	Sirolimus	Wyeth	Not available
Rebetol®	Ribavirin	Schering	800-656-9485

Medications and the Sponsoring Programs' Contact Numbers cont.

BRAND NAME	GENERIC NAME	SPONSORING COMPANY	TELEPHONE
Recombinate®	Recombinant antihemophilic factor	Baxter	800-548-4448
ReFacto®	Antihemophilic factor	Wyeth	Not available
Reglan®	Metoclopramide	Whitehall-Robins	Not available
Relafen®	Nabumetone	GSK	866-728-4368
Relenza®	Zanamavir	GSK	866-728-4368
Relpax®	Eletriptan	Pfizer	800-717-6005
Remeron®	Mirtazapine	Organon	973-325-5273
Remicade®	Infliximab	Centocor	866-489-5957
Reminyl®	Galantamine	Centocor	866-489-5957
Renagel®	Sevelamer	Genzyme	800-638-8299
Reopro®	Abciximab	Lilly	800-545-6962
Repronex®	Menotropins for injection	Ferring	Not available
Requip®	Ropinirole	GSK	866-728-4368
Rescriptor®	Delavirdine	Pfizer	800-717-1761
RespiGam®	Respiratory syncytial virus immune globulin	MedImmune	Not available
Restasis®	Cyclosporine ophthalmic	Allergan	800-553-6783
Restoril®	Temazepam	Novartis	Not available
Retavase®	Reteplase	Centocor	866-489-5957
Retrovir®	Zidovudine	GSK	866-728-4368
Reyataz™	Atazanavir	BMS	800-272-4878
Rhinocort Aqua®	Budesonide	AstraZeneca	800-424-3727

Medications and the Sponsoring Programs' Contact Numbers cont.

BRAND NAME	GENERIC NAME	SPONSORING COMPANY	TELEPHONE
Rilutek®	Riluzole	Aventis	800-459-7599
Risperdal®	Risperidone	Janssen	800-652-6227, ext.1
Ritalin LA®	Methylphenidate hydrochloride	Novartis	800-277-2254
Rituxan®	Rituximab	Genentech	800-530-3083
RMS®	Rectal morphine	Upsher-Smith	800-654-2299
Robinul®	Glycopyrrolate	First Horizon	800-869-4514
Rythmol SR®	Propafenone	Abbott	Not available
Salagen®	Pilocarpine	MGI	888-743-5711
Sandimmune®	Cyclosporine	Novartis	800-277-2254
Sectral®	Acebutolol	ESP Pharma	908-850-6192
Semprex®-D	Acrivastine/pseudoephedrine	Celltech	866-523-3994
Septra®	Trimethoprim/ sulfamethoxazole	Monarch	Not available
Serevent®	Salmeterol xinafoate	GSK	866-728-4368
Seroquel®	Quetiapine	AstraZeneca	800-424-3727
Sinemet®	Carbidopa/levodopa	BMS	800-736-0003
Sinequan®	Doxepin	Pfizer	800-717-6005
Singulair®	Montelukast	Merck	800-727-5400
Slo-Niacin®	Controlled-release niacin	Upsher-Smith	800-654-2299
Solaquin Forte®	Hydroquinone with sunscreen	Valeant	800-556-1937, ext. 4
Soma®	Carisoprodol	Wallace	Not available
Somavert®	Pegvisomant	Pfizer	800-645-1280

Medications and the Sponsoring Programs' Contact Numbers cont.

BRAND NAME	GENERIC NAME	SPONSORING COMPANY	TELEPHONE
Spiriva®	Tiotropium	BI	800-556-8317
SSKI®	Potassium iodide	Upsher Smith	800-654-2299
Stelazine®	Trifluoperazine	GSK	866-728-4368
Stromectal®	Ivermectin	Merck	Not available
Sular®	Nisoldipine	First Horizon	800-869-4514
Sulfacet®	Sulfacetamide sodium/ sulfur lotion	Dermik	866-268-7326
Sumycin®	Tetracycline	Par	Not available
Sustiva®	Efavirenz	BMS	800-272-4878
Symmetrel®	Amantadine	Endo	908-684-5799
Synagis®	Palivizumab	MedImmune	877-480-8082
Synalar®	Fluocinolone acetonide solution	Medicis	800-711-0811
Synthroid®	Levothyroxine	Abott	800-222-6885
Synvisc®	Hylan G-F 20	Wyeth	Not available
Syprine®	Trientine	Merck	800-727-5400
Tabloid®	Thioguanine	GSK	866-265-6491
Tagamet®	Cimetidine	GSK	866-728-4368
Tambocor®	Flecainide	3M	800-328-0255
Tamiflu®	Oseltamivir	Roche	800-285-4484
Tapazole®	Methimazole	King	877-546-5332
Targretin®	Bexarotene	Ligand	877-654-4263
Tarka®	Trandolapril/verapamil	Abbott	800-222-6885

Medications and the Sponsoring Programs' Contact Numbers cont.

BRAND NAME	GENERIC NAME	SPONSORING COMPANY	TELEPHONE
Taxol®	Paclitaxel	BMS	800-272-4878
Taxotere®	Docetaxel	Aventis	800-221-4025
Tegretol®	Carbamazepine	Novartis	800-277-2254
Temodar®	Temozolomide	Schering	800-521-7157
Temovate®	Clobetasol propionate cream	GSK	866-728-4368
Tensilon®	Edrophonium	Valeant	Not available
Tequin®	Gatifloxacin	BMS	800-736-0003
Terramycin®	Oxytetracycline	Pfizer	Not available
Teslac®	Testolactone	BMS	800-272-4878
Tessalon®	Benzonatate	Forest	800-851-0758
Teveten®	Eprosartan	Biovail	866-268-7325
Thalitone®	Chlorthalidone	King	877-546-5332
Thalomid®	Thalidomide	Celgene	888-423-5436
Theochron®	Theophylline	Forest	800-851-0758
Theolair™	Theophylline	3M	Not available
Thorazine®	Chlorpromazine	GSK	866-728-4368
Thyrel® TRH	Protirelin	Ferring	Not available
Thyrolar®	Liotrix	Forest	800-851-0758
Tiazac®	Diltiazem	Forest	800-851-0758
Ticlid®	Ticlopidine	Roche	800-285-4484
Tikosyn™	Dofetilide	Pfizer	Not available
Tilade®	Nedocromil	King	877-546-5332
Timentin®	Ticarcillin/clavulanate	GSK	866-728-4368

Medications and the Sponsoring Programs' Contact Numbers cont.

BRAND NAME	GENERIC NAME	SPONSORING COMPANY	TELEPHONE
Timoptic®	Timolol maleate ophthalmic solution	Merck	800-994-2111
TNKase®	Tenecteplase	Genentech	800-530-3083
Topamax®	Topiramate	Ortho-McNeil	800-577-3788
Topicort®	Desoximetasone cream	Medicis	800-711-0811
Toprol-XL®	Metoprolol succinate	AstraZeneca	800-424-3727
Trandate®	Labetalol	Prometheus	Not available
Travatan®	Travoprost	Alcon	800-222-8103, ext. 1
Trecator®	Ethionamide	Wyeth	800-568-9938
Triaz®	Benzoyl peroxide gel	Medicis	800-550-5115
Tricor®	Fenofibrate	Abbott	800-222-6885
Trileptal®	Oxcarbazepine	Novartis	800-277-2254
Trimox®	Amoxicillin	BMS	800-736-0003
Triphasil®	Levonorgestrel/ ethinyl estradiol	Wyeth	Not available
Trivora-28®	Levonorgestrel/ ethinyl estradiol	Watson	Not available
Trizivir®	Abacavir/lamivudine/ zidovudine	GSK	866-728-4368
Truvada®	Emtricitabine/tenofovir	Gilead	Not available
Tussionex® Pennkinetic®	Hydrocodone polistirex/ chlorpheniramine polistirex	Celltech	866-523-3994
Tylenol® with codeine	Acetaminophen with codeine	Ortho-McNeil	800-865-7211

Medications and the Sponsoring Programs' Contact Numbers cont.

BRAND NAME	GENERIC NAME	SPONSORING COMPANY	TELEPHONE
Tylox®	Acetaminophen/oxycodone	Ortho-McNeil	800-865-7211
Ultracet®	Tramadol/acetaminophen	Ortho-McNeil	800-577-3788
Ultram®	Tramadol	Ortho-McNeil	800-577-3788
Ultrase®	Amylase/lipase/protease	Axcan Scandipharm	800-472-2634
Ultravate™	Halobetasol propionate cream	BMS	800-736-0003
Univasc®	Moexipril	Schwarz	Not available
Urso 250™	Ursodiol	Axcan Scandipharm	866-292-2679
Vagifem®	Estradiol vaginal	Novo Nordisk	866-668-6336
Valium®	Diazepam	Roche	800-285-4484
Valtrex®	Valacyclovir	GSK	866-728-4368
Vancocin®	Vancomycin	Lilly	800-545-6962
Vasodilan®	Isoxsuprine	BMS	800-736-0003
Vasotec®	Enalapril	Merck	Not available
Venofer®	Iron sucrose injection	American Regent	800-282-7712
Ventolin®	Albuterol aerosol inhaler	GSK	866-728-4368
VePesid®	Etoposide	BMS	800-272-4878
Verelan®	Verapamil	Schwarz	Not available
Viagra®	Sildenafil	Pfizer	800-717-6005
Vibramycin®	Doxycycline	Pfizer	800-717-6005
Vicodin®	Hydrocodone/acetaminophen	Abbott	800-222-6885
Videx®	Didanosine	BMS	800-272-4878

Medications and the Sponsoring Programs' Contact Numbers cont.

BRAND NAME	GENERIC NAME	SPONSORING COMPANY	TELEPHONE
Viokase®	Amylase/lipase/protease	Axcan Scandipharm	866-292-2679
Viracept®	Nelfinavir	Pfizer	888-777-6637
Viramune®	Nevirapine	BI	800-556-8317
Virazole®	Ribavirin inhalation solution	Valeant	800-556-1937, ext. 4
Viread®	Tenofovir	Gilead	800-226-2056
Viroptic®	Trifluridine	King	877-546-5332
Visken®	Pindolol	Novartis	Not available
Vistaril®	Hydroxyzine	Pfizer	800-717-6005
Vistide®	Cidofovir injection	Gilead	800-226-2056
Volmax®	Albuterol inhaler	Muro	800-225-0974, ext. 3
Voltaren®	Diclofenac	Novartis	800-277-2254
Vumon®	Teniposide injection	BMS	800-272-4878
Vytone®	Hydrocortisone/ iodoquinol cream	Dermik	866-268-7326
Vytorin™	Ezetimibe/simvastatin	Merck/Schering	800-347-7503
Welchol®	Colesevelam	Sankyo	866-268-7327
Wellbutrin®	Bupropion	GSK	866-728-4368
WinRho SDF®	Rho (D) immune globulin	Nabi	800-789-209
Xanax®	Alprazolam	Pfizer	800-717-6005
Xenical®	Orlistat	Roche	800-285-4484
Xolair®	Omalizumab	Genentech	Not available
Xyrem®	Sodium oxybate	Orphan	866-997-3688

Medications and the Sponsoring Programs' Contact Numbers cont.

BRAND NAME	GENERIC NAME	SPONSORING COMPANY	TELEPHONE
Zantac®	Ranitidine	GSK	866-728-4368
Zarontin®	Ethosuximide	Pfizer	800-717-6005
Zaroxolyn®	Metolazone	Celltech	866-523-3994
Zebeta®	Bisoprolol	Wyeth	Not available
Zerit®	Stavudine	BMS	800-736-0003
Zestril®	Lisinopril	AstraZeneca	Not available
Zestoretic®	Lisinopril/HCTZ	AstraZeneca	Not available
Zetia™	Ezetimibe	Merck/Schering	800-347-7503
Ziac®	Bisoprolol/HCTZ	Wyeth	Not available
Ziagen®	Abacavir	GSK	866-728-4368
Zinacef®	Cefuroxime	GSK	866-728-4368
Zithromax®	Azithromycin	Pfizer	800-717-6005
Zocor®	Simvastatin	Merck	800-727-5400
Zofran®	Ondansetron	GSK	866-728-4368
Zoladex®	Goserelin acetate implant	AstraZeneca	800-424-3727
Zoloft®	Sertraline	Pfizer	800-717-6005
Zometa®	Zoledronic	Novartis	800-282-7630 ext. 2, then 2
Zomig®	Zolmitriptan	AstraZeneca	800-424-3727
Zonegran®	Zonisamide	Elan	866-347-3185
Zovirax®	Acyclovir	GSK	866-268-7325
Zyban®	Bupropion	GSK	866-728-4368

Medications and the Sponsoring Programs' Contact Numbers cont.

BRAND NAME	GENERIC NAME	SPONSORING COMPANY	TELEPHONE
Zyloprim®	Allopurinol	Faro	Not available
Zyprexa®	Olanzapine	Lilly	800-488-2133
Zyrtec®	Cetirizine	Pfizer	800-717-6005
Zyvox®	Linezolid	Pfizer	800-717-1761

Not available: Drug is not available in a pharmaceutical assistance program.
Note: BI is Boehringer Ingelheim; BMS is Bristol-Myers Squibb; ECR is ECR Pharmaceuticals; GSK is Glaxo Smith Kline; MGI is MGI Pharmaceuticals; P&G is Proctor & Gamble.

A FINAL THOUGHT,
A FINAL STRATEGY

Drug Smarts
and Drug Safety

W E AMERICANS are the most medicated folks on the planet. More than 40 percent of all Americans take at least one prescription medication, and more than 80 percent of those ages 65 and over take prescription drugs. Even for the young, those under age 18, nearly one-quarter take at least one prescription drug. Our consumption to take prescription drugs seems insatiable—now drugs are being prescribed for "social anxiety disorder" (shyness) and "adult attention deficit disorder" (impulsivity or distractibility).

During your doctor appointment, ask a different question. Don't "ask your doctor" questions suggested by television advertisements about Viagra® or Levitra® for erectile dysfunction, about the "purple pill" that extinguishes the smoldering fires of reflux, or about medication to kill that toenail scourge, "Digger the Dermatophyte." Instead, ask your doctor if there are any medications that you can *quit* taking.

Doctors are quick to prescribe medications; after all, we want to help our patients, and there are hundreds of drugs available. The United States is one of only two countries in the world (New Zealand is the other) that allows direct marketing of prescription drugs to consumers—and the billions of dollars spent on marketing work. My patients frequently request a prescription of a medication that was advertised on television. Even more money is spent by drug companies to market pharmaceuticals to physicians, expounding on the benefits of new prescription drugs while encouraging us to prescribe them.

Sometimes a doctor may start a medication for a temporary problem but then never stop prescribing it. This happens not uncommonly with medications used to treat heartburn, when a change in dietary patterns might suffice. Perhaps you had a drug started during a hospitalization for a good reason; however, now you are home and may no longer require it. The doctor who prescribed the medication in the hospital may be different from your regular doctor and not aware of all of the medications, vitamins, and herbal supplements that you are taking at home. If so, ask your doctor at your next visit if you still need that medication.

The Risks of Taking More than One Medication

When you take a drug, you incur risks from side effects in addition to the benefits you derive from treatment. These risks increase greatly as the number of drugs you take increases due to interactions among the different drugs, as well as additive side effects. Many drugs affect the metabolism of other drugs or share similar side effects. Simply put, the more drugs you take, the more likely you are to suffer from a side effect.

The elderly are particularly at risk from taking multiple medications, given their diminished ability to metabolize drugs as a result of the reduced kidney and liver function associated with aging. Frail, gaunt patients may overdose by taking a typical dosage. Ask your doctor if a lower dose can be prescribed; this is an effective way to reduce your chances of drug side effects.

Occasionally, doctors may treat one medication's side effect by prescribing yet another medication. The best-selling medication to treat hypertension is Norvasc®, which can cause swelling of the feet as a side effect. Despite the edema being the side effect of a drug, a doctor may treat the patient's swollen feet with two other medications: a diuretic to decrease the swelling and potassium replacement. Replacing Norvasc® with a different drug to lower the elevated blood pressure—without producing swelling—is a far better solution.

Many herbal supplements interact with prescription drugs. Unlike prescription drugs, which are carefully regulated by the FDA, herbal supplements face no such requirements. Supplements are particularly worrisome for those taking anticoagulants. Vitamin E and ginkgo can make bleeding more likely; ginseng may make the blood of those taking Coumadin® (warfarin) thicker.

Drug interactions have become so commonplace that they are topical in popular movies. In the hit movie *Something's Gotta Give* Jack Nicholson's character is asked if he takes Viagra®. He denies taking it until the doctor informs him of its side effect when taken with nitroglycerin. Jack immediately reconsiders his denial, then rips the nitroglycerin drip out of his vein. Tagamet®, Zantac®, and Pepcid® change the pH of the stomach and can affect other drugs' absorption, as well as the metabolism of many drugs. Muscle aches, and even toxicity, are more likely among those taking statins such as Zocor® when they are also taking the blood pressure medication Calan® (verapamil) or the antibiotic Biaxin® (clarithromycin).

Drug Recalls

Unfortunately, some side effects are not recognized for a very long time and may result in heart attacks or even death. Severe side effects are detected by individual cases' being reported to the FDA or by clinical trials performed after the drug has been released. More than a dozen drugs have been withdrawn from the U.S. market since 1997 due to safety concerns. Most of these drugs were on the market for several years before they were withdrawn, and tens of millions of Americans have taken these popular medications. The recent voluntary recall of Vioxx® by Merck and other recalls will illustrate several important points and help to debunk four myths.

Drugs Recalled by the FDA Since 1997

YEARS APPROVED, THEN RECALLED	BRAND (GENERIC) NAMES	CONDITION TREATED	REASON RECALLED
1997–2001	Baycol® (cerivastatin)	Elevated cholesterol	Risk of developing rhabdomyolysis, a potentially fatal muscle injury

1999–2001	Raplon® (rapacuronium)	Anesthetic	Risk of developing bronchospasm, an inability to breathe normally
1993–2000	Propulsid® (cisapride)	Nighttime heartburn	Risk of developing fatal heart rhythm abnormalities
1997–2000	Rezulin® (troglitazone)	Type 2 diabetes	Risk of severe liver toxicity
1962–2000*	(phenylpropanolamine)	Congestion from colds	Risk of bleeding in the brain
2000–2000	Lotronex® (alosetron)	Irritable bowel syndrome in women	Risk of intestinal damage or ruptured bowels
1988–1999	Hismanal® (astemizole)	Allergies and runny nose	Risk of developing fatal heart rhythm abnormalities
1997–1999	Raxar® (grepafloxacin)	Infection	Risk of developing fatal heart rhythm abnormalities
1985–1998	Seldane® (terfenadine)	Allergies and runny nose	Risk of developing fatal heart rhythm abnormalities
1997–1998	Posicor® (mibefradil)	High blood pressure	Risk of numerous dangerous drug interactions
1997–1998	Duract® (bromfenac)	Acute pain	Risk of severe liver damage
1993–1997	Redux® (dexfenfluramine)	Obesity	Risk of developing heart valve abnormalities
1973–1997	Pondimin® (fenfluramine)	Obesity	Risk of developing heart valve abnormalities

This list is modified from the FDA website, www.fda.gov/fdac/features/2002/chrtWithdrawals.html.
*Phenylpropanolamine, a popular generic drug, was in use prior to 1962, when an amendment to food and drug laws required a review of the effectiveness of this and other drugs while they remained on the market. This popular drug was an ingredient in many over-the-counter cold preparations before the FDA acted to withdraw it from the market.

Benadryl® is an old and effective antihistamine used to treat seasonal allergies; however, it had the undesirable side effect of making many people drowsy. In the 1980s, two popular antihistamines became available as nonsedating antihistamines. Although they were not stronger than Benadryl®, Seldane® and Hismanal® did not cause sleepiness and thus were widely prescribed. Both drugs were on the market for more than a decade before they were associated with increased risk of serious heart rhythm abnormality and withdrawn—obviously a very long delay for such an important side effect to be noted in widely prescribed drugs.

In 2001, Baycol®, a medication used to lower cholesterol levels, was withdrawn abruptly after the drug was discovered to be causing a form of severe muscle weakness called rhabdomyolysis. This potentially fatal condition occurred primarily in patients treated with a higher dose of Baycol® in conjunction with another cholesterol-lowering medication, Lopid®. Baycol® was available on the U.S. market for four years before this lethal drug interaction became widely known.

The end of the twentieth century saw the development and promotion of a new, novel class of drugs deemed the "superaspirins." These COX-2 (cyclooxygenase enzyme-2) inhibitors, Celebrex®, Vioxx®, and Bextra®, quickly became among the best-selling drugs in the United States. This was not in small part due to their television ads, such as the one with Dorothy Hamill ice-skating effortlessly while the lyrics "It's a beautiful morning" played in the background.

These drugs are used for treating pain from arthritis. Unlike the older NSAIDs (nonsteroidal anti-inflammatory drugs) Advil® and Naprosyn®, the newer Bextra® Celebrex®, and Vioxx®, were not supposed to cause as much stomach irritation. As previously discussed, the older NSAIDs nonselectively inhibited the cyclooxygenase enzyme, leading to stomach discomfort in a number of patients. By inhibiting only the COX-2 enzyme, it was felt, these new drugs would be safer. None of the drugs provides more pain relief than the older medications in large clinincal trials.

In clinical trials, Vioxx® was the only drug among the new COX-2 inhibitors able to prove that it caused less stomach irritation than the older drug Naprosyn®. Alarmingly, the VIGOR study, published in *The New England Journal of Medicine* on November 23, 2000, also revealed that those taking Vioxx® had more heart attacks than those taking Naprosyn®. The study raised the question of whether Vioxx® was causing heart attacks or whether Naprosyn® had an added benefit of reducing heart attacks that had not previously been noted.

A subsequent study of 2,600 patients with colon polpys compared Vioxx® to a placebo—not to Naprosyn®. The safety monitoring of the study conclusively showed an increased risk for heart attacks and strokes among those taking Vioxx®. Merck withdrew Vioxx® from the U.S. market on September 30, 2004, and the withdrawal has heightened concerns about drug safety. These cases provide several important messages.

Myth 1: Drugs taken for minor ailments have minor, if any, side effects. Drugs used for relatively benign conditions—allergies and joint pain—can have lethal side effects. Taking the drug was far worse than the disease for those who suffered side effects. It has been estimated that 80 million people have taken Vioxx® and that more than 100,000 heart attacks may have been caused by the drug which was widely prescribed from 1999 to 2004. Remember, just because the condition that you are taking the drug for is benign does not mean that the drug is benign.

Myth 2: If the drug has been approved by the FDA and available for years, it must be safe. In most cases of recalled drugs, it takes years to determine that there is an increased risk. Seldane® and Hismanal® were on the market for more than a decade before being withdrawn. The FDA is under pressure to approve new drugs to benefit the public, and a consequence is that extensive, long-term safety studies are not being performed. The general method that the FDA uses to evaluate drugs for safety problems involves "watchful waiting," in which physicians report adverse effects after the drug is released, drug companies report safety monitoring, and published data are reviewed. The study precipitating the withdrawal of Vioxx® was a large one that tested more than two thousand patients. Even with that large number of patients, the problem was not detected until eighteen months later. If the study had lasted one year or had involved fewer patients, the increased risk of heart attack among those taking Vioxx® might not have been detected, and Vioxx® might have been felt to be a safe drug based on the large study.

Myth 3: Newer drugs are always better than older drugs. "New" does not always mean "improved." Newer drugs are not always safer than older ones, and in some cases they may be more harmful than the drugs they are replacing. Almost every drug is tested against a placebo in clinical trials rather than being compared to the drug that it is replacing. Generally, it is not possible to truly know if the new drug is safer than an older medication. Merck was unusual in that it tested Vioxx® against Naprosyn®, a drug it was intended to replace.

Myth 4: Mixing medications is safe. Drugs that are safe to take individually may become life-threatening when taken with other medications, and drug interactions increase with the number of drugs you take. In the case of Baycol®, the drug interaction with Lopid® was fatal, because the drugs' metabolism affected each other. In the cases of Propulsid®, Hismanal®, and Seldane®, these drugs caused QT prolongation. The QT interval is the time that it takes the heart to repolarize after beating. Prolongation of the QT interval can provoke arrhythmias in patients taking other drugs that prolonged the QT interval or who had low potassium levels.

Take Better Care of Yourself

Think back to your high school graduation and imagine that you received a brand-new car as a graduation present. It didn't happen for me, either, but imagine it nonetheless. It is a beautiful car and will take you wherever you want to go—with one catch. The car must last you all your life, and you cannot get another car. If the car breaks down, you are stuck and can't go anywhere. What would you do to maintain your car? Wouldn't you make sure it was properly serviced, had regularly scheduled oil changes, and kept in optimal working order? How good are you at giving your body, the vehicle that takes you everywhere, the care it needs?

Do you smoke? If you smoke, you are much more likely to need drugs for your lungs and heart and to fight cancer. Smoking is the most preventable underlying cause of premature death in the United States and is responsible for 440,000 deaths annually. There is no other consumer product that will kill you when used as directed, nor

BE DRUG SMART: FIVE EASY QUESTIONS TO ASK YOUR DOCTOR:

1) Why am I taking this drug? A surprising number of patients can't name which drugs they are taking or why they are taking them. You should bring a list of your drugs and all pill bottles to each doctor's visit. Some patients have difficulty with medical terminology. Don't worry, so do most first-year medical students and pharmacy students. Ask your doctor or nurse to help you make a medication list with the brand name, generic name, instructions on when to take the medication, and purpose of the medication. Make sure you know which drugs you are taking and why you are taking them.

2) Do I need all these drugs? This is the single best question to ask your doctor to see if some medications can be stopped. The best time to ask this question is after you have made lifestyle changes: If you have lost weight, you might not need the same medications for your hypertension and diabetes. If you have recently quit smoking, perhaps some of your lung medications can be stopped. And be sure to remind your doctor about medications you started taking in the hospital; once you are home, perhaps they can be stopped.

3) Will this drug interact with any of the other medications or supplements I am taking? Many supplements interact with drugs so make sure to tell your doctor what you are taking on a regular or occasional basis. And, of course, medications often interact with each other, so make sure your doctor knows about any over-the-counter pills you take or drugs prescribed by another doctor. Remember that unlike drugs, the FDA does not regulate supplements. Any claims of benefits from taking the supplement or even the actual contents of the supplement may not be accurate.

4) What are the major side effects, how often do patients get them, and is there a safer drug available? All drugs have side effects but some are more common or more serious than others. Express your concerns to your doctor, who may be able to help you find an alternative.

5) Are any of the strategies in this book appropriate for me? Make sure your doctor knows that you need help in making your prescription drugs more affordable and accessible. Proactive patients save more money than passive patients.

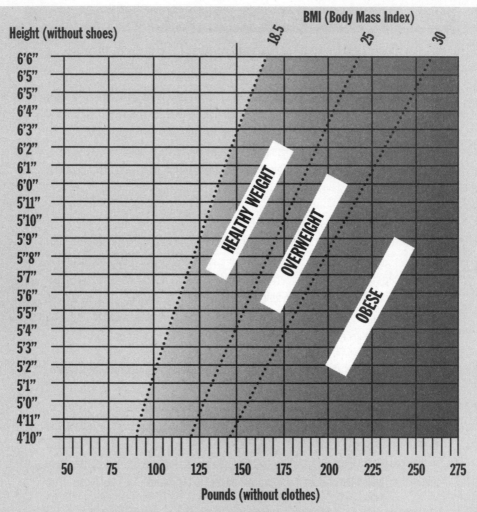

BMI measures weight in relation to height. The BMI ranges shown above are for adults. They are not exact ranges of healthy and unhealthy weights. However, they show that health risk increases at higher levels of overweight and obesity. Even within the healthy BMI range, weight gains can carry health risks for adults.

Directions: Find your weight on the bottom of the graph. Go straight up from that point until you come to the line that matches your height. Then look to find your weight group.

Healthy Weight: BMI from 18.5 up to 25 refers to a healthy weight.
Overweight: BMI from 25 up to 30 refers to overweight.
Obese: BMI 30 or higher refers to obesity. Obese persons are also overweight.

is there any pill that will help your longevity as much as not smoking.

Are you medically overweight or obese? Check the body mass index table from the National Institutes of Health to see if you are. Weighing too much leads to hypertension, diabetes, and high cholesterol levels. In fact, obesity is the second most common preventable cause of premature death in the United States and is responsible for about 400,000 premature deaths annually. Eating less, losing ten or more pounds if you are overweight, and doing a simple exercise program, such as walking for thirty minutes three times a week, will greatly impact your health—and reduce your prescription drug cost. I have been able to discontinue drugs for many patients who have substantially changed their lifestyle. Not smoking, losing weight, greatly reducing dietary salt and fat, and regularly exercising will not totally eliminate the need for drugs in most cases, but it can certainly reduce the number and dosages of drugs that are needed.

Karen is a patient who was able to stop her medications because of lifestyle changes. I met 67-year-old Karen in May, when she was on medications for elevated blood pressure and cholesterol. She was frustrated about her weight, and her BMI was in the obese range. Having tried diets in addition to phen-fen before it was removed from the market, she was open to trying something new. After testing Karen's heart, I asked her to go to the local cardiac rehabilitation program for its wellness program. It is more difficult to lose weight without regular exercise, and exercise builds up additional muscle mass. Since a pound of muscle burns more calories than a pound of fat, increasing your muscle mass helps by increasing your resting metabolism. I also asked Karen to be a vegetarian for one month and see how much weight she lost. She was already eating in a reasonably "healthy" manner, avoiding fatty foods, sweets, and breads. We discussed the fact that that the new federal guidelines encourage fruits and vegetables and one easy way of increasing your intake of them is to be a vegetarian. Five months later, a buffer Karen returned, off her medications and about twenty pounds lighter. She kept with the fitness program and decided to remain vegetarian. She felt great—better than she had felt in years—and she even thanked me for giving her back her health.

In conclusion, review your medications with your doctor and ask if you can reduce or stop any of them. Do not reduce or stop any drugs without your doctor's approval. You will be more likely to reduce the amount of medications you need if you adopt a more healthful lifestyle. You'll feel better, too.

PART II

Drugs for Less Listing

T HIS FINAL SECTION summarizes the information presented in the preceding chapters to give you practical suggestions on reducing *your* cost of many expensive brand-name drugs. Each page lists a brand-name drug, as well as the monthly and annual cost of taking a commonly prescribed dose of that drug. Drugs that are combinations of two medications in one tablet are listed on the same pages as the major component drugs.

In most cases, the cost per tablet of each listed medication exceeds $1, and the annual cost of taking one drug exceeds $500. More than twenty of these drugs have an estimated annual cost exceeding $1,000. Taking several of these drugs simultaneously will break almost anyone's budget. The list contains more than one hundred commonly prescribed brand-name medications used to treat chronic illnesses such as hypertension, diabetes, heartburn, elevated cholesterol levels, depression, erectile dysfunction, and arthritis. These are among the most prescribed drugs in the United States, and the most difficult to afford.

To reduce your overall cost, four to seven methods to obtain your drugs for less cost are presented for each drug. If your prescription drug is not included in this list, check the index for the brand and generic names and refer to those pages for cost-cutting ideas. Any cost-cutting techniques need to be discussed with your doctor, who understands the particulars of your care. We may suggest slicing tablets, for instance, but your doctor would then need to write you a prescription for a higher dosage. A lower-cost drug may possibly be substituted for the listed medication; however, your doctor would need to carefully consider the substitution. As always, you need to follow your doctor's recommendations.

Medications are listed on individual pages so that you can photocopy the pertinent pages, then discuss ways to reduce your prescription drug cost with your doctor and pharmacist. The price of each drug was taken from the Costco and FamilyMeds online pharmacy's websites, accessed in late 2004 and early 2005. These websites are convenient to check and offer low prices. The best way for you to reduce your cost of medications is to become better informed and more proactive. Your doctor will be aware of your apprehension about rising prescription drug costs only if you express your concerns about them.

It is impossible to receive high quality medical care without access to prescription drugs. Many of the benefits of modern treatments are bestowed by the careful use of prescription drugs, and medications remain an important adjunct to surgery. I hope that the information contained in *Drugs for Less* has made your prescription drugs more affordable and thus more accessible. Please email any comments or concerns to me at DrMichael@drmichael.com. My website, www.drmichael.com, contains additional information and a message board for discussion. Any ideas that you have to reduce cost can be shared there. I wish you good health and the benefits of affordable prescription drugs.

ACCOLATE® (ZAFIRLUKAST)

Accolate® is a leukotriene receptor blocker used to treat patients with asthma. A typical dose for Accolate® is 20 mg twice daily, and the price for sixty tablets is about $80. The annual cost for this medication is about $960. To decrease your cost, consider the following alternatives:

1. Ask your doctor for samples.
2. Purchase larger quantities at a discount pharmacy such as those listed in Strategy 2.
3. Investigate the government programs listed in Strategy 6, including Medicaid, the Veterans Health Administration, and state assistance programs.
4. If you are taking a dose of 10 mg twice daily, ask your doctor if you may purchase 20 mg tablets of Accolate® and use a pill cutter to slice the tablet into two 10 mg parts.
5. Contact the AstraZeneca Foundation Patient Assistance Program by telephoning 800-424-3727.

ACCUPRIL® (QUINAPRIL)
ACCURETIC® (QUINAPRIL/HCTZ)

Accupril® is an ACE inhibitor used to treat patients with high blood pressure or congestive heart failure. Accuretic® is a combination tablet that has Accupril® plus a diuretic. A typical dose of Accupril® is 20 mg daily, and the price of thirty tablets is $38.09. The annual cost of this medication is about $450. A typical dose of Accuretic® is 20/12.5 mg; the price of thirty tablets is $43.09 and the annual cost of this dose is about $510. To decrease the cost, consider the following alternatives:

1. Ask your doctor for samples.
2. Purchase larger quantities at a discount pharmacy such as those listed in Strategy 2.
3. Investigate the government programs listed in Strategy 6, including Medicaid, the Veterans Health Administration, and state assistance programs.
4. Ask your doctor if you may purchase 40 mg tablets of Accupril® and use a pill cutter to slice the tablet into two 20 mg parts. Accuretic® may also be sliced with your doctor's approval.
5. Ask your doctor if you may substitute generic quinapril or quinapril/HCTZ for brand-name Accupril® or Accuretic®.
6. Ask your doctor if you may substitute generic captoril, enalapril, or lisinopril for brand-name Accupril®. These generic medications are also ACE inhibitors with similar indications.
7. Ask your doctor if substituting a generic diuretic such as HCTZ or chlorthalidone along with a generic ACE inhibitor instead of Accuretic® is appropriate.
8. Contact the Pfizer Connection to Care Program by telephoning 800-707-8990.

ACEON® (PERINDOPRIL)

Aceon® is an ACE inhibitor used to treat patients with high blood pressure. A typical dose of Aceon® is 4 mg daily, and the price of thirty tablets is $48.69. The annual cost of this medication is about $580. To decrease your cost, consider the following alternatives:

1. Ask your doctor for samples.
2. Purchase larger quantities at a discount pharmacy such as those listed in Strategy 2.
3. Investigate the government programs listed in Strategy 6, including Medicaid, the Veterans Health Administration, and state assistance programs.
4. Ask your doctor if you may purchase 8 mg tablets of Aceon® and use a pill cutter to slice the tablet into two 4 mg parts.
5. Ask your doctor if you may substitute generic captopril, enalapril, or lisinopril for brand-name Aceon®. These generic medications are also ACE inhibitors with similar indications.
6. Contact the Solvay Pharmaceuticals, Inc. Patient Assistance Program by telephoning 800-256-8918.

ACIPHEX® (RABEPRAZOLE)

Aciphex® is a proton pump inhibitor used to treat heartburn, ulcers, and acid reflux. A typical dose of Aciphex® is 20 mg daily, and the price of thirty tablets is $123.37. Although it generally should not be taken on a daily basis for a year, the annual cost of this medication, if taken daily, would be about $1,480. To decrease your cost, consider the following alternatives:

1. Ask your doctor for samples.
2. Purchase larger quantities at a discount pharmacy such as those listed in Strategy 2.
3. Investigate the government programs listed in Strategy 6, including Medicaid, the Veterans Health Administration, and state assistance programs.
4. Ask your doctor if Prilosec® or generic omperazole 20 mg daily would be an acceptable substitute for Aciphex®. Prilosec® is available without a prescription at much less cost.
5. Ask your doctor if an H2 blocker like generic cimetidine, ranitidine, or famotidine would be an acceptable substitute for Aciphex®. These medications, which work differently than proton pump inhibitors, are available without a prescription at much less cost.
6. Contact the Janssen Patient Assistance Program by telephoning 800-523-5870.

ACTONEL® (RISEDRONATE)

Actonel® is a bisphosphonate used to treat osteoporosis. A typical dose of Actonel® is 35 mg weekly, and the price of four tablets is $64.77. The annual cost of this medication is about $840. To decrease your cost, consider the following alternatives:

1. Ask your doctor for samples.
2. Purchase larger quantities at a discount pharmacy such as those listed in Strategy 2.
3. Investigate the government programs listed in Strategy 6, including Medicaid, the Veterans Health Administration, and state assistance programs.
4. Ask your doctor if other treatments for osteoporosis, such as vitamin D and calcium supplementation in addition to exercise would be an acceptable substitute for Actonel®.
5. Contact the Procter & Gamble Patient Assistance Program by telephoning 800-830-9049.

ACTOS® (PIOGLITAZONE)

Actos® is a thiazolidinedione drug used to treat diabetic patients. A typical dose of Actos® is 30 mg daily, and the price of thirty tablets is $156.79. The annual cost of this medication is about $1,880. To decrease your cost, consider the following alternatives:

1. Ask your doctor for samples.
2. Purchase larger quantities at a discount pharmacy such as those listed in Strategy 2.
3. Investigate the government programs listed in Strategy 6, including Medicaid, the Veterans Health Administration, and state assistance programs.
4. Ask your doctor if you may purchase 45 mg tablets of Actos® and use a pill cutter to slice the tablet into two 22.5 mg parts. Slicing is infrequently done as 22.5 mg is not a standard dosage.
5. Ask your doctor if you may substitute generic glyburide, or glipizide for brand-name Actos®. These diabetes medications are sulfonylurea drugs that work differently than Actos® and may not be appropriate.
6. Ask your doctor if Avandia® 4 mg would be an acceptable substitute for Actos®. Avandia® is a thiazolidinedione drug with similar properties that may be available at less cost than Actos®. Avandia® tablets may also be sliced into two halves with a pill cutter.
7. Contact the Takeda Pharmaceuticals Patient Assistance Program by telephoning 800-830-9159.

ADVAIR™ DISKUS® (SALMETEROL/FLUTICASONE)

Advair™ Diskus® is an inhaler containing a corticosteroid and a beta₂agonist drug, and it is used to treat patients with asthma. A typical dose for Advair™ Diskus® is one unit twice daily, and the price for sixty units of the 0.25mg/0.05mg /inhalation dose is $140.77. The annual cost of this medication is about $1,690. To decrease your cost, consider the following alternatives:

1. Ask your doctor for samples.
2. Purchase larger quantities at a discount pharmacy such as those listed in Strategy 2.
3. Investigate the government programs listed in Strategy 6, including Medicaid, the Veterans Health Administration, and state assistance programs.
4. Contact the GlaxoSmithKline Bridges to Access Program by having an advocate telephone 866-728-4368.

ALLEGRA® (FEXOFENADINE)
ALLEGRA D® (FEXOFENADINE/PSEUDOEPHEDRINE)

Allegra® is a nonsedating antihistamine used to treat seasonal allergy symptoms, including watery eyes and runny nose. Allegra D® is an extended release combination tablet of Allegra® and pseudoephedrine, a decongestant available without prescription. A typical dose of Allegra® is 180 mg daily, and the price of thirty tablets is $67.29. Although it generally should not be taken on a daily basis for a year, the annual cost of this medication would be about $800. A typical dose of Allegra D® is 60 mg/120mg daily, and the price of thirty tablets is $40.97 with an annual cost of about $490. To decrease your cost, consider the following alternatives:

1. Ask your doctor for samples.
2. Purchase larger quantities at a discount pharmacy such as those listed in Strategy 2.
3. Investigate the government programs listed in Strategy 6, including Medicaid, the Veterans Health Administration, and state assistance programs.
4. Ask your doctor if you may substitute Claritin® or generic loratadine 10 mg daily for Allegra®. Both Claritin® and generic loratadine are available without a prescription at much less cost.
5. Ask your doctor if substituting over-the-counter pseudoephedrine and Allegra® or over-the-counter pseudoephedrine and loratadine for Allegra D® is appropriate. Because pseudoephedrine is an ingredient used in the illegal manufacturing of methamphetamine, sales of this medication may be limited.
6. Contact the Aventis Patient Assistance Program by telephoning 800-221-4025.

ALTACE® (RAMIPRIL)

Altace® is an ACE inhibitor used to treat patients with high blood pressure or congestive heart failure. A typical dose of Altace® is 5 mg daily, and the price of thirty capsules is $40.59. The annual cost of this medication is about $490. To decrease your cost, consider the following alternatives:

1. Ask your doctor for samples.
2. Purchase larger quantities at a discount pharmacy such as those listed in Strategy 2.
3. Investigate the government programs listed in Strategy 6, including Medicaid, the Veterans Health Administration, and state assistance programs.
4. Ask your doctor if you may substitute generic captopril, enalapril, or lisinopril for brand-name Altace®. These generic medications are also ACE inhibitors with similar indications.
5. Contact the King Kare Patient Assistance Program by telephoning 877-546-5332.

AMARYL® (GLIMEPIRIDE)

Amaryl® is a sulfonylurea drug used to treat diabetic patients. A typical dose of Amaryl® is 2 mg daily, and the price of thirty tablets is $20.17. The annual cost of this medication is about $240. To decrease your cost, consider the following alternatives:

1. Ask your doctor for samples.
2. Purchase larger quantities at a discount pharmacy such as those listed in Strategy 2.
3. Investigate the government programs listed in Strategy 6, including Medicaid, the Veterans Health Administration, and state assistance programs.
4. Ask your doctor if you may purchase 4 mg tablets of Amaryl® and use a pill cutter to slice the tablet into two 2 mg parts.
5. Ask your doctor if you may substitute generic glyburide, or glipizide for brand-name Amaryl®. These generic medications are sulfonylurea drugs with similar indications.
6. Contact the Aventis Patient Assistance Program by telephoning 800-221-4025.

AMBIEN® (ZOLPIDEM)

Ambien® is a non-benzodiazepine hypnotic drug used to treat insomnia. A typical dose of Ambien® is 5 mg at bedtime, and the price of thirty tablets is $69.27. Although Ambien® should not be taken every day, the annual cost of this medication would be about $830. To decrease your cost, consider the following alternatives

1. Ask your doctor for samples.
2. Purchase larger quantities at a discount pharmacy such as those listed in Strategy 2.
3. Investigate the government programs listed in Strategy 6, including Medicaid, the Veterans Health Administration, and state assistance programs.
4. Purchase 10 mg tablets of Ambien® and use a pill cutter to slice the tablet into two 5 mg parts *if your doctor feels this is appropriate.*
5. Ask your doctor if you may substitute generic temazepam (Restoril®), or triazolam (Halcion®) for brand-name Ambien®. These generic medications are benzodiazepine drugs used to treat insomnia.

ATACAND® (CANDESARTAN)
ATACAND HCT® (CANDESARTAN/HCTZ)

Atacand® is an angiotensin receptor blocker used to treat patients with high blood pressure. Atacand HCT® is a combination tablet that contains Atacand® and a diuretic. A typical dose of Atacand® is 16 mg daily, and the price of thirty tablets is $47.57. The annual cost of this medication is about $570. The price of thirty tablets of a typical dose of Atacand HCT® 16/12.5 mg is $64.67, and the annual cost of this dose is about $770. To decrease your cost, consider the following alternatives:

1. Ask your doctor for samples.
2. Purchase larger quantities at a discount pharmacy such as those listed in Strategy 2.
3. Investigate the government programs listed in Strategy 6, including Medicaid, the Veterans Health Administration, and state assistance programs.
4. Ask your doctor if you may purchase 32 mg tablets of Atacand® and use a pill cutter to slice the tablet into two 16 mg parts. Atacand HCT® may also be sliced with your doctor's approval.
5. Ask your doctor if you may substitute generic captopril, enalapril, or lisinopril for brand-name Atacand®. These generic medications are ACE inhibitors and have similar indications to those of angiotensin receptor blockers. Some patients can't take ACE inhibitors because they develop a cough.
6. Ask your doctor if substituting a generic diuretic such as HCTZ or chlorthalidone and taking it with a generic ACE inhibitor is appropriate instead of taking Atacand HCT®.
7. Contact the AstraZeneca Foundation Patient Assistance Program by telephoning 800-424-3727.

ATROVENT® (IPRATROPIUM)

Atrovent® MDI (metered dose inhaler) is an inhaler containing an anticholinergic bronchodilator used to treat patients with COPD. A typical dose for Atrovent® MDI is two puff four times daily, and the price for one inhaler is $60.67. The annual cost of this medication is about $730. To decrease your cost, consider the following alternatives:

1. Ask your doctor for samples.
2. Purchase larger quantities at a discount pharmacy such as those listed in Strategy 2.
3. Investigate the government programs listed in Strategy 6, including Medicaid, the Veterans Health Administration, and state assistance programs.
4. Ask your doctor if you may purchase a nebulizer and use generic ipratopium solution as an aerosolized solution rather than using the more expensive MDI. Medicare may pay for the cost of a home nebulizer and the ipratropium solution. Although there is a generic ipratopium solution, there is not a generic ipratopium MDI.
5. Contact the Boehringer Ingelheim Care Foundation Patient Assistance Program by telephoning 800-556-8317.

AUGMENTIN® (AMOXICILLIN/CLAVULANATE)

Augmentin® is an antibiotic frequently used to treat bacterial infections. A typical dose of Augmentin® involves taking 250 mg/125 mg tablets three times daily for one week to ten days, and the price of thirty tablets is $92.79. To decrease your cost, consider the following alternatives:

1. Ask your doctor for samples.
2. Purchase larger quantities at a discount pharmacy such as those listed in Strategy 2.
3. Investigate the government programs listed in Strategy 6, including Medicaid, the Veterans Health Administration, and state assistance programs.
4. Ask your doctor if taking a different type of antibiotic, such as generic amoxicillin or trimethoprim/sulfamethoxazole for brand-name Augmentin® is appropriate. Those who are allergic to penicillin should not take Augmentin® or amoxicillin and those who are allergic to sulfa should not take trimethoprim/sulfamethoxazole.
5. Contact the GlaxoSmithKline Bridges to Access Program by having an advocate telephone 866-728-4368.

AVANDIA® (ROSIGLITAZONE)

Avandia® is a thiazolidinedione drug used to treat diabetic patients. A typical dose of Avandia® is 4 mg daily, and the price of thirty tablets is $85.69. The annual cost of this medication is about $1,030. To decrease your cost, consider the following alternatives:

1. Ask your doctor for samples.
2. Purchase larger quantities at a discount pharmacy such as those listed in Strategy 2.
3. Investigate the government programs listed in Strategy 6, including Medicaid, the Veterans Health Administration, and state assistance programs.
4. Ask your doctor if you may purchase 8 mg tablets of Avandia® and use a pill cutter to slice the tablet into two 4 mg parts.
5. Ask your doctor if you may substitute generic glyburide or glipizide for brand-name Avandia®. These diabetes medications are sulfonylurea drugs that work differently from Avandia®.
6. Contact the GlaxoSmithKline Bridges to Access program by having an advocate telephone 866-728-4368.

AVAPRO® (IRBESARTAN)
AVALIDE® (IRBESARTAN/HCTZ)

Avapro® is an angiotensin receptor blocker used to treat patients with high blood pressure. Avalide® is a combination tablet that contains Avapro® and a diuretic. A typical dose of Avapro® is 150 mg daily, and the price of thirty tablets is $48.89. The annual cost of this medication is about $580. The price of thirty tablets of a typical dose of Avalide® 150/12.5 mg is $63.99, and the annual cost of this dose is about $760. To decrease your cost, consider the following alternatives:

1. Ask your doctor for samples.
2. Purchase larger quantities at a discount pharmacy such as those listed in Strategy 2.
3. Investigate the government programs listed in Strategy 6, including Medicaid, the Veterans Health Administration, and state assistance programs.
4. Ask your doctor if you may purchase 300 mg tablets of Avapro® and use a pill cutter to slice the tablet into two 150 mg parts. Avalide® may also be sliced with your doctor's approval.
5. Ask your doctor if you may substitute generic captopril, enalapril, or lisinopril for brand-name Avapro® These generic medications are ACE inhibitors and have similar indications to those of angiotensin receptor blockers. Some patients can't take ACE inhibitors because they develop a cough.
6. Ask your doctor if substituting a generic diuretic such as HCTZ or chlorthalidone and taking it with a generic ACE inhibitor is appropriate instead of taking Avalide®.
7. Contact the Bristol-Myers Squibb Patient Assistance Foundation by telephoning 800-736-0003.

AVELOX® (MOXIFLOXACIN)

Avelox® is an antibiotic used to treat bacterial infections. A typical dose of Avelox® is 400 mg tablets once daily for one week, and the price of seven tablets is about $65. To decrease your cost, consider the following alternatives:

1. Ask your doctor for samples.
2. Purchase larger quantities at a discount pharmacy such as those listed in Strategy 2.
3. Investigate the government programs listed in Strategy 6, including Medicaid, the Veterans Health Administration, and state assistance programs.
4. Ask your doctor if you may substitute generic ciprofloxacin for brand-name Avelox®; both are quinolone antibiotics.
5. Ask your doctor if substituting a different type of antibiotic, such as generic amoxicillin or trimethoprim/sulfamethoxazole for brand-name Avelox® is appropriate. Those who are allergic to penicillin cannot take amoxicillin and those who are allergic to sulfa cannot take trimethoprim/sulfamethoxazole.
6. Contact the Bayer Patient Assistance Program by telephoning 800-998-9180.

BENICAR™ (OLMESARTAN)
BENICAR HCT™ (OLMESARTAN/ HCTZ)

Benicar™ is an angiotensin receptor blocker used to treat patients with high blood pressure. Benicar HCT™ is a combination tablet that contains Benicar™ and a diuretic. A typical dose of Benicar™ is 20 mg daily, and the price of thirty tablets is $50.69. The annual cost of this medication is about $610. The price of thirty tablets of a typical dose of Benicar HCT™ 40/12.5 mg is $55.59, and the annual cost of this dose is about $670. To decrease your cost, consider the following alternatives:

1. Ask your doctor for samples.
2. Purchase larger quantities at a discount pharmacy such as those listed in Strategy 2.
3. Investigate the government programs listed in Strategy 6, including Medicaid, the Veterans Health Administration, and state assistance programs.
4. Ask your doctor if you may purchase 40 mg tablets of Benicar™ and use a pill cutter to slice the tablet into two 20 mg parts. Benicar HCT™ may also be sliced with your doctor's approval.
5. Ask your doctor if you may substitute generic captopril, enalapril, or lisinopril for brand-name Benicar™. These generic medications are ACE inhibitors and have similar indications to angiotensin receptor blockers. Some patients can't take ACE inhibitors because they develop a cough.
6. Ask your doctor if substituting a generic diuretic such as HCTZ or chlorthalidone and take it with a generic ACE inhibitor is appropriate instead of taking Benicar HCT™.
7. Contact the Sankyo Pharma Open Care Program by telephoning 866-268-7327, ext. 1.

BEXTRA® (VALDECOXIB)

Bextra® decreases inflammation by inhibiting the cyclooxygenase-2 (COX-2) enzyme and is used to treat patients with arthritis and muscle aches. A typical dose of Bextra® is 10 mg daily, and the price of thirty tablets is $90.27. Although it frequently is not taken on a daily basis for a year, the annual cost of this medication would be about $1,080. To decrease your cost, consider the following alternatives:

1. Ask your doctor for samples.
2. Purchase larger quantities at a discount pharmacy such as those listed in Strategy 2.
3. Investigate the government programs listed in Strategy 6, including Medicaid, the Veterans Health Administration, and state assistance programs.
4. Ask your doctor if you may purchase 20 mg tablets of Bextra® and use a pill cutter to slice the tablet into two 10 mg parts.
5. Ask your doctor if you may substitute a generic NSAIDs—such as ibuprofen or naproxen—for Bextra®. These medications are available without a prescription at much less cost. NSAIDs work differently from COX-2 inhibitors, and side effects may prohibit their use by some patients.
6. Contact the Pfizer Connection to Care Program by telephoning 800-707-8990.

BIAXIN® (CLARITHROMYCIN)

Biaxin® is an antibiotic frequently used to treat bacterial infections. A typical dose of Biaxin® involves taking 250 mg tablets twice daily for one week to ten days, and the price of twenty tablets is $86.52. Biaxin® XL is an extended release form of Biaxin®. To decrease your cost, consider the following alternatives:

1. Ask your doctor for samples.
2. Purchase larger quantities at a discount pharmacy such as those listed in Strategy 2.
3. Investigate the government programs listed in Strategy 6, including Medicaid, the Veterans Health Administration, and state assistance programs.
4. Ask your doctor if taking a different type of antibiotic, such as generic amoxicillin or trimethoprim/sulfamethoxazole for brand-name Biaxin® is appropriate. Those who are allergic to penicillin cannot take amoxicillin and those who are allergic to sulfa cannot take trimethoprim/sulfamethoxazole.
5. Contact the Abbott Laboratories Patient Assistance Program by telephoning 800-222-6885.

CELEBREX® (CELECOXIB)

Celebrex® decreases inflammation by inhibiting the cyclooxygenase-2 (COX-2) enzyme and is used to treat patients with arthritis and muscle aches. A typical dose of Celebrex® is 200 mg daily, and the price of thirty capsules is $93.42. Although it frequently is not taken on a daily basis for a year, the annual cost of this medication is about $1,120. To decrease your cost, consider the following alternatives:

1. Ask your doctor for samples.
2. Purchase larger quantities at a discount pharmacy such as those listed in Strategy 2.
3. Investigate the government programs listed in Strategy 6, including Medicaid, the Veterans Health Administration, and state assistance programs.
4. Ask your doctor if you may substitute a generic NSAID—such as ibuprofen or naproxen—for Celebrex®. These medications are available without a prescription at much less cost. NSAIDs work differently from COX-2 inhibitors, and side effects may prohibit their use by some patients.
5. Contact the Pfizer Connection to Care Program by telephoning 800-707-8990.

CELEXA® (CITALOPRAM)

Celexa® is a selective serotonin reuptake inhibitor (SSRI) antidepressant used to treat patients with major depression. A typical dose of Celexa® is 20 mg daily, and the price of thirty tablets is $73.99. The annual cost of this medication is about $890. To decrease your cost, consider the following alternatives:

1. Ask your doctor for samples.
2. Purchase larger quantities at a discount pharmacy such as those listed in Strategy 2.
3. Investigate the government programs listed in Strategy 6, including Medicaid, the Veterans Health Administration, and state assistance programs.
4. Purchase 40 mg tablets of Celexa® and use a pill cutter to slice the tablet into two 20 mg parts *if your doctor feels this is appropriate.*
5. Ask your doctor if you may substitute generic citalopram for brand-name Celexa®.
6. Contact the Forest Pharmaceuticals Patient Assistance Program by telephoning 800-851-0758.

CIALIS® (TADALAFIL)

Cialis® is used to treat men with erectile dysfunction. A typical dose of Cialis® is 10 mg and the price of thirty tablets is about $280. To decrease your cost, consider the following alternatives:

1. Ask your doctor for samples.
2. Purchase larger quantities at a discount pharmacy such as those listed in Strategy 2.
3. Investigate the government programs listed in Strategy 6, including Medicaid, the Veterans Health Administration, and state assistance programs.
4. Ask your doctor if you may purchase 20 mg tablets of Cialis® and use a pill cutter to slice the tablet into two 10 mg parts.

CIPRO® (CIPROFLOXACIN)

Cipro® is an antibiotic frequently used to treat bacterial infections. A typical dose of Cipro® involves taking 500 mg tablets twice daily for one week to ten days, and the price of twenty tablets is $106.33. To decrease your cost, consider the following alternatives:

1. Ask your doctor for samples.
2. Purchase larger quantities at a discount pharmacy such as those listed in Strategy 2.
3. Investigate the government programs listed in Strategy 6, including Medicaid, the Veterans Health Administration, and state assistance programs.
4. Purchase generic ciprofloxacin rather than brand-name Cipro®.
5. Ask your doctor if substituting a different type of antibiotic, such as generic amoxicillin or trimethoprim/sulfamethoxazole for brand-name Cipro® is appropriate. Those who are allergic to penicillin cannot take amoxicillin and those who are allergic to sulfa cannot take trimethoprim/sulfamethoxazole.
6. Contact the Bayer Patient Assistance Program by telephoning 800-998-9180.

CLARINEX® (DESLORATADINE)

Clarinex® is a nonsedating antihistamine used to treat seasonal allergy symptoms, including watery eyes and runny nose. A typical dose of Clarinex® is 5 mg daily, and the price of thirty tablets is $65.67. Although it generally should not be taken on a daily basis for a year, the annual cost of this medication is about $790. To decrease your cost, consider the following alternatives:

1. Ask your doctor for samples.
2. Purchase larger quantities at a discount pharmacy such as those listed in Strategy 2.
3. Investigate the government programs listed in Strategy 6, including Medicaid, the Veterans Health Administration, and state assistance programs.
4. Ask your doctor if Claritin® or generic loratadine 10 mg daily would be an acceptable substitute for Clarinex®. Both Claritin® and generic loratadine are available without a prescription at much less cost.
5. Contact the Schering Laboratories Patient Assistance Program by telephoning 800-656-9485.

COMBIVENT® (ALBUTEROL/IPRATOPIUM)

Combivent® MDI (metered dose inhaler) is an inhaler containing beta₂agonist and anticholinergic bronchodilator drugs used to treat patients with COPD. A typical dose for Combivent® MDI is two puff four times daily, and the price for one inhaler is $67.77. The annual cost of this medication is about $810. To decrease your cost, consider the following alternatives:

1. Ask your doctor for samples.
2. Purchase larger quantities at a discount pharmacy such as those listed in Strategy 2.
3. Investigate the government programs listed in Strategy 6, including Medicaid, the Veterans Health Administration, and state assistance programs.
4. Ask your doctor if you may purchase a nebulizer and use generic albuterol and ipratopium solution as an aerosolized solution rather than using the more expensive MDI. Medicare may pay for a home nebulizer as well as the generic albuterol and ipratropium solution. Although there is a generic ipratopium solution, there is not a generic ipratopium MDI.
5. Contact the Boehringer Ingelheim Care Foundation Patient Assistance Program by telephoning 800-556-8317.

COREG® (CARVEDILOL)

Coreg® is a beta-blocker with special properties that is used to treat patients with congestive heart failure. A typical dose of Coreg® is 12.5 mg twice daily, and the price of a one-month supply of sixty tablets is about $104. The annual cost of this medication is about $1,250. To decrease your cost, consider the following alternatives:

1. Ask your doctor for samples.
2. Purchase larger quantities at a discount pharmacy such as those listed in Strategy 2.
3. Investigate the government programs listed in Strategy 6, including Medicaid, the Veterans Health Administration, and state assistance programs.
4. Ask your doctor if you may purchase 25 mg tablets of Coreg® and use a pill cutter to slice the tablet into two 12.5 mg parts.
5. Ask your doctor if you may substitute generic metoprolol tartate or brand-name Toprol XL® (metoprolol succinate) for Coreg®. Both generic metoprolol tartate and brand-name Toprol XL® are suitable for slicing if you doctor approves.
6. Contact the GlaxoSmithKline Bridges to Access program by having an advocate telephone 866-728-4368.

COUMADIN® (WARFARIN)

Coumadin® is a blood thinner that inhibits vitamin K dependant clotting factors and is used to treat patients with atrial fibrillation, prosthetic heart valves, and other conditions. A typical dose of Coumadin® is 5 mg once daily, and the price of a one-month supply of thirty tablets is about $23.39. The annual cost of this medication is about $280. To decrease your cost, consider the following alternatives:

1. Ask your doctor for samples.
2. Purchase larger quantities at a discount pharmacy such as those listed in Strategy 2.
3. Investigate the government programs listed in Strategy 6, including Medicaid, the Veterans Health Administration, and state assistance programs.
4. Ask your doctor if you may substitute generic warfarin for Coumadin®.
5. Contact the Bristol-Myers Squibb Patient Assistance Foundation by telephoning 800-736-0003.

COZAAR® (LOSARTAN)
HYZAAR® (LOSARTAN/HCTZ)

Cozaar® is an angiotensin receptor blocker used to treat patients with high blood pressure. Hyzaar® is a combination tablet that contains Cozaar® and a diuretic. A typical dose of Cozaar® is 50 mg daily, and the price of thirty tablets is $44.97. The annual cost of this medication is about $540. The price of thirty tablets of a typical dose of Hyzaar® 50/12.5 mg is nearly identical at $45.47. To decrease your cost, consider the following alternatives:

1. Ask your doctor for samples.
2. Purchase larger quantities at a discount pharmacy such as those listed in Strategy 2.
3. Investigate the government programs listed in Strategy 6, including Medicaid, the Veterans Health Administration, and state assistance programs.
4. Ask your doctor if you may purchase 100 mg tablets of Cozaar® and use a pill cutter to slice the tablet into two 50 mg parts. Hyzaar® may also be sliced with your doctor's approval.
5. Ask your doctor if you may substitute generic captopril, enalapril, or lisinopril for brand-name Cozaar®. These generic medications are ACE inhibitors and have similar indications to those of angiotensin receptor blockers. Some patients can't take ACE inhibitors because they develop a cough.
6. Ask your doctor if substituting a generic diuretic such as HCTZ or chlorthalidone and taking it with a generic ACE inhibitor is appropriate instead of taking Hyzaar®.
7. Contact the Merck Patient Assistance Program by telephoning 800-727-5400.

CRESTOR® (ROSUVASTATIN)

Crestor® is a statin used to lower cholesterol levels, particularly the LDL cholesterol that clogs arteries. A typical dose of Crestor® is 10 mg daily, and the price of thirty tablets is $76.87. The annual cost of this medication is about $920. To decrease your cost, consider the following alternatives:

1. Ask your doctor for samples.
2. Purchase larger quantities at a discount pharmacy such as those listed in Strategy 2.
3. Investigate the government programs listed in Strategy 6, including Medicaid, the Veterans Health Administration, and state assistance programs.
4. Ask your doctor if you may purchase 20 mg tablets of Crestor® and use a pill cutter to slice the tablet into two 10 mg parts.
5. Ask your doctor if taking generic lovastatin would be an acceptable substitute for Crestor®. Generic lovastatin may be sliced into two parts with your doctor's approval.
6. Contact the AstraZeneca Foundation Patient Assistance Program by telephoning 800-424-3727.

DIFLUCAN® (FLUCONAZOLE)

Diflucan® is an antifungal used to treat Candida infections. A typical dose of Diflucan® used to treat oral Candida infections is to take two 100 mg tablets on the first day then to take one 100 mg tablet daily for a minimum of three weeks. The price for thirty tablets is $278.09. To decrease your cost, consider the following alternatives:

1. Ask your doctor for samples.
2. Purchase larger quantities at a discount pharmacy such as those listed in Strategy 2.
3. Investigate the government programs listed in Strategy 6, including Medicaid, the Veterans Health Administration, and state assistance programs.
4. Ask your doctor if you may substitute generic flucanazole for brand-name Diflucan®.
5. Contact the Pfizer Connection to Care Program by telephoning 800-707-8990.

DIOVAN® (VALSARTAN)
DIOVAN HCT® (VALSARTAN/HCTZ)

Diovan® is an angiotensin receptor blocker used to treat patients with high blood pressure. Diovan HCT® is a combination tablet that contains Diovan® and a diuretic. A typical dose of Diovan® is 80 mg daily, and the price of thirty tablets is $47.69. The annual cost of this medication is about $570. The price of thirty tablets of a typical dose of Diovan HCT® 80/12.5 mg is $52.59, for an annual cost of about $630. To decrease your cost, consider the following alternatives:

1. Ask your doctor for samples.
2. Purchase larger quantities at a discount pharmacy such as those listed in Strategy 2.
3. Investigate the government programs listed in Strategy 6, including Medicaid, the Veterans Health Administration, and state assistance programs.
4. Ask your doctor if you may purchase 160 mg tablets of Diovan® and use a pill cutter to slice the tablet into two 80 mg parts. Diovan HCT® may also be sliced with your doctor's approval.
5. Ask your doctor if you may substitute generic captopril, enalapril, or lisinopril for brand-name Diovan®. These generic medications are ACE inhibitors and have similar indications to those of angiotensin receptor blockers. Some patients can't take ACE inhibitors because they develop a cough.
6. Ask your doctor if substituting a generic diuretic such as HCTZ or chlorthalidone and taking it with a generic ACE inhibitor is appropriate instead of taking Diovan HCT®.
7. Contact the Novartis Patient Assistance Program by telephoning 800-277-2254.

EFFEXOR XR® (VENLAFAXINE)

Effexor XR® is a serotonin and norepinephrine reuptake inhibitor (SSNRI) antidepressant used to treat patients with major depression. A typical dose of Effexor XR® is 75 mg daily, and the price of thirty tablets is $89.67. The annual cost of this medication is about $1,080. To decrease your cost, consider the following alternatives:

1. Ask your doctor for samples.
2. Purchase larger quantities at a discount pharmacy such as those listed in Strategy 2.
3. Investigate the government programs listed in Strategy 6, including Medicaid, the Veterans Health Administration, and state assistance programs.
4. Contact the Wyeth Patient Assistance Program by telephoning 800-568-9938.

EVISTA® (RISEDRONATE)

Evista® is a selective estrogen receptor modulator (SERM) used to prevent postmenopausal osteoporosis. A typical dose of Evista® is 60 mg daily, and the price of thirty tablets is $78.87. The annual cost of this medication is about $950. To decrease your cost, consider the following alternatives:

1. Ask your doctor for samples.
2. Purchase larger quantities at a discount pharmacy such as those listed in Strategy 2.
3. Investigate the government programs listed in Strategy 6, including Medicaid, the Veterans Health Administration, and state assistance programs.
4. Ask your doctor if other treatments for osteoporosis, such as vitamin D and calcium supplementation in addition to exercise, would be an acceptable substitute for Evista®.
5. Contact the Lilly Cares Patient Assistance Program by telephoning 800-545-6962.

FOSAMAX® (RISEDRONATE)

Fosamax® is a bisphosphonate used to treat osteoporosis. A typical dose of Fosamax® is 70 mg weekly, and the price of four tablets is $68.09. The annual cost of this medication is about $890. To decrease your cost, consider the following alternatives:

1. Ask your doctor for samples.
2. Purchase larger quantities at a discount pharmacy such as those listed in Strategy 2.
3. Investigate the government programs listed in Strategy 6, including Medicaid, the Veterans Health Administration, and state assistance programs.
4. Ask your doctor if other treatments for osteoporosis, such as vitamin D and calcium supplementation in addition to exercise would be an acceptable substitute for Fosamax®.
5. Contact the Merck Patient Assistance Program by telephoning 800-727-5400.

FLOMAX® (TAMSULOSIN)

Flomax® is an alpha$_{A1}$ adrenoreceptor blocker used to treat patients with benign prostatic hypertrophy. A typical dose of Flomax® is 0.4mg once daily, and the price for thirty capsules is $53.39. The annual cost for this medication is about $640. To decrease your cost, consider the following alternatives:

1. Ask your doctor for samples.
2. Purchase larger quantities at a discount pharmacy such as those listed in Strategy 2.
3. Investigate the government programs listed in Strategy 6, including Medicaid, the Veterans Health Administration, and state assistance programs.
4. Ask your doctor if taking generic Hytrin® (terazosin) would be an acceptable substitute. Hytrin® works differently than Flomax® and lowers the blood pressure so it may not be an acceptable substitute for you.
5. Contact the Boehringer Ingelheim Care Foundation Patient Assistance Program by telephoning 800-556-8317.

FLONASE® (FLUTICASONE)

Flonase® is a nasal spray containing a corticosteroid used to treat patients with allergic rhinitis. A typical dose for Flonase® is two sprays in each nostril daily, and the price for one nasal pump bottle is $61.99. To decrease your cost, consider the following alternatives:

1. Ask your doctor for samples.
2. Purchase larger quantities at a discount pharmacy such as those listed in Strategy 2.
3. Investigate the government programs listed in Strategy 6, including Medicaid, the Veterans Health Administration, and state assistance programs.
4. Ask your doctor if an over-the-counter brand-name Afrin® (oxymetazoline) or its generic substitute is an appropriate substitute. These medications are not corticosteroids and provide relief from nasal congestion by a different mechanism.
5. Contact the GlaxoSmithKline Bridges to Access Program by having an advocate telephone 866-728-4368.

FLOVENT® (FLUTICASONE)

Flovent® MDI (metered dose inhaler) contains a corticosteroid used to treat patients with asthma. A typical dose for Flovent® MDI is two puff twice daily, and the price for one inhaler is $79.67. The annual cost of this medication is about $950. To decrease your cost, consider the following alternatives:

1. Ask your doctor for samples.
2. Purchase larger quantities at a discount pharmacy such as those listed in Strategy 2.
3. Investigate the government programs listed in Strategy 6, including Medicaid, the Veterans Health Administration, and state assistance programs.
4. Contact the GlaxoSmithKline Bridges to Access Program by having an advocate telephone 866-728-4368.

FLOXIN® (OFLOXACIN)

Floxin® is an antibiotic used to treat bacterial infections. A typical dose of Floxin® is 400 mg tablets twice daily for ten days, and the price of twenty tablets is about $125. To decrease your cost, consider the following alternatives:

1. Ask your doctor for samples.
2. Purchase larger quantities at a discount pharmacy such as those listed in Strategy 2.
3. Investigate the government programs listed in Strategy 6, including Medicaid, the Veterans Health Administration, and state assistance programs.
4. Ask your doctor if you may substitute generic ofloxacin for brand-name Floxin®.
5. Ask your doctor if substituting a different type of antibiotic, such as generic amoxicillin or trimethoprim/sulfamethoxazole for brand-name Floxin® is appropriate. Those who are allergic to penicillin cannot take amoxicillin and those who are allergic to sulfa cannot take trimethoprim/sulfamethoxazole.
6. Contact the Ortho McNeil Patient Assistance Program by having an advocate telephone 800-577-3788.

GLUCOPHAGE® XR (METFORMIN)

Glucophage® XR is a biguanide drug used to treat diabetic patients. A typical dose of Glucophage® XR is 500 mg twice daily, and the price for sixty tablets is about $50. The annual cost for this medication is about $600. To decrease your cost, consider the following alternatives:

1. Ask your doctor for samples.
2. Purchase larger quantities at a discount pharmacy such as those listed in Strategy 2.
3. Investigate the government programs listed in Strategy 6, including Medicaid, the Veterans Health Administration, and state assistance programs.
4. Ask your doctor if you may purchase 1,000 mg tablets of generic metformin and use a pill cutter to slice the tablet into two 500 mg parts. Glucophage® XR is not suitable for slicing.
5. Ask your doctor if you may substitute generic metformin extended release for brand name Glucophage® XR.
6. Contact the Bristol-Myers Squibb Pharmaceutical Assistance Foundation by having an advocate telephone 800-736-0003.

GLUCOTROL XL® (GLIPIZIDE)

Glucotrol XL® is a sulfonylurea drug used to treat diabetic patients. A typical dose of Glucotrol XL® is 5 mg daily, and the price for thirty tablets is $15.59. The annual cost for this medication is about $190. To decrease your cost, consider the following alternatives:

1. Ask your doctor for samples.
2. Purchase larger quantities at a discount pharmacy such as those listed in Strategy 2.
3. Investigate the government programs listed in Strategy 6, including Medicaid, the Veterans Health Administration, and state assistance programs.
4. Ask your doctor if you may purchase 10 mg tablets of glipizide and use a pill cutter to slice the tablet into two 5 mg parts. Glucotrol XL® is not suitable for slicing.
5. Ask your doctor if you may substitute generic extended release glipizide for brand name Glucotrol XL®.
6. Contact the Pfizer Connection to Care Program by having an advocate telephone 800-707-8990.

GLUCOVANCE® (METFORMIN/GLYBURIDE)

Glucovance® is a combination tablet that contains two different types of medications used to treat diabetic patients. A typical dose of Glucovance® is 2.5 mg/500 mg daily, and the price for thirty tablets is $32.49. The annual cost for this medication is about $390. To decrease your cost, consider the following alternatives:

1. Ask your doctor for samples.
2. Purchase larger quantities at a discount pharmacy such as those listed in Strategy 2.
3. Investigate the government programs listed in Strategy 6, including Medicaid, the Veterans Health Administration, and state assistance programs.
4. Ask your doctor if you may substitute generic metformin/glyburide combination tablets for brand-name Glucovance®.
5. Ask your doctor if you may substitute separate doses of generic metformin and generic glyburide for brand-name Glucovance®.
6. Contact the Bristol-Myers Squibb Pharmaceutical Assistance Foundation by having an advocate telephone 800-736-0003.

IMITREX® (SUMATRIPTAN)

Imitrex® is a 5-hydroxytryptamine$_1$ receptor agonist used to treat patients with migraine headaches. A typical dose for Imitrex® is 50 mg, and the price for nine tablets is $154.29. To decrease your cost, consider the following alternatives:

1. Ask your doctor for samples.
2. Purchase larger quantities at a discount pharmacy such as those listed in Strategy 2.
3. Investigate the government programs listed in Strategy 6, including Medicaid, the Veterans Health Administration, and state assistance programs.
4. Purchase 100 mg tablets of Imitrex® and use a pill cutter to slice the tablet into two 50 mg parts *if your doctor feels this is appropriate.*
5. Contact the GlaxoSmithKline Pharmaceutical Assistance Program by having an advocate telephone 866-728-4368.

INDERAL® LA (PROPRANOLOL)

Inderal® LA is a beta-blocker used to treat patients with high blood pressure. A typical dose of Inderal® LA is 80 mg daily, and the price for thirty tablets is $45.27. The annual cost for this medication is about $540. To decrease your cost, consider the following alternatives:

1. Ask your doctor for samples.
2. Purchase larger quantities at a discount pharmacy such as those listed in Strategy 2.
3. Investigate the government programs listed in Strategy 6, including Medicaid, the Veterans Health Administration, and state assistance programs.
4. Ask your doctor if you may take generic propranolol instead of Inderal® LA. Generic propranolol must be taken twice daily.
5. Contact the Wyeth Patient Assistance Program by having an advocate telephone 800-568-9938.

LESCOL XL® (FLUVASTATIN)

Lescol XL® is a statin used to lower cholesterol levels, particularly the LDL cholesterol that clogs arteries. A typical dose of Lescol XL® is 80 mg daily, and the price of thirty tablets is $66.67. The annual cost of this medication is about $800. To decrease your cost, consider the following alternatives:

1. Ask your doctor for samples.
2. Purchase larger quantities at a discount pharmacy such as those listed in Strategy 2.
3. Investigate the government programs listed in Strategy 6, including Medicaid, the Veterans Health Administration, and state assistance programs.
4. Ask your doctor if generic lovastatin would be an acceptable substitute for Lescol XL®. Generic lovastatin may be sliced into two parts with your doctor's approval. Lescol XL® is not suitable for slicing.
5. Ask your doctor if taking a sliced tablet of the more potent Lipitor® or Crestor® would be an acceptable substitute.
6. Contact the Novartis Patient Assistance Program by having an advocate telephone 800-277-2254.

LEVAQUIN® (LEVOFLOXACIN)

Levaquin® is an antibiotic used to treat bacterial infections. A typical dose of Levaquin® is 500 mg once daily for seven days, and the price of seven tablets is about $70. To decrease your cost, consider the following alternatives:

1. Ask your doctor for samples.
2. Purchase larger quantities at a discount pharmacy such as those listed in Strategy 2.
3. Investigate the government programs listed in Strategy 6, including Medicaid, the Veterans Health Administration, and state assistance programs.
4. Ask your doctor if you may substitute generic ciprofloxacin for brand-name Levaquin®; both are quinolone antibiotics.
5. Ask your doctor if substituting a different type of antibiotic, such as generic amoxicillin or trimethoprim/sulfamethoxazole for brand-name Levaquin® is appropriate. Those who are allergic to penicillin cannot take amoxicillin and those who are allergic to sulfa cannot take trimethoprim/sulfamethoxazole.
6. Contact the Ortho McNeil Patient Assistance Program by having an advocate telephone 800-577-3788.

LEVITRA® (VARDENAFIL)

Levitra® is used to treat men with erectile dysfunction. A typical dose of Levitra® is 10 mg, and the price of thirty tablets is $264.87. To decrease your cost, consider the following alternatives:

1. Ask your doctor for samples.
2. Purchase larger quantities at a discount pharmacy such as those listed in Strategy 2.
3. Investigate the government programs listed in Strategy 6, including Medicaid, the Veterans Health Administration, and state assistance programs.
4. Ask your doctor if you may purchase 20 mg tablets of Levitra® and use a pill cutter to slice the tablet into two 10 mg parts.

LEXAPRO® (ESCITALOPRAM)

Lexapro® is a selective serotonin reuptake inhibitor, SSRI, antidepressant used to treat patients with major depression. A typical dose of
Lexapro® is 10 mg daily, and the price of thirty tablets is $64.89. The
annual cost of this medication is about $780. To decrease your cost,
consider the following alternatives:

1. Ask your doctor for samples.
2. Purchase larger quantities at a discount pharmacy such as those
   listed in Strategy 2.
3. Investigate the government programs listed in Strategy 6, including
   Medicaid, the Veterans Health Administration, and state assistance
   programs.
4. Purchase 20 mg tablets of Lexapro® and use a pill cutter to slice
   the tablet into two 10 mg parts *if your doctor feels this is appropriate.*
5. Contact the Forest Pharmaceuticals Patient Assistance Program by
   having an advocate telephone 800-851-0758.

LIPITOR® (ATORVASTATIN)

Lipitor® is a statin used to lower cholesterol levels, particularly the LDL cholesterol that clogs arteries. A typical dose of Lipitor® is 10 mg daily, and the price of thirty tablets is $71.47. The annual cost of this medication is about $860. To decrease your cost, consider the following alternatives:

1. Ask your doctor for samples.
2. Purchase larger quantities at a discount pharmacy such as those listed in Strategy 2.
3. Investigate the government programs listed in Strategy 6, including Medicaid, the Veterans Health Administration, and state assistance programs.
4. Ask your doctor if you may purchase 20 mg tablets of Lipitor® and use a pill cutter to slice the tablet into two 10 mg parts.
5. Ask your doctor if generic lovastatin would be an acceptable substitute for Lipitor®. The generic lovastatin may be sliced into two parts with your doctor's approval.
6. Contact the Pfizer Connection to Care Program by having an advocate telephone 800-707-8990.

LOTENSIN® (BENAZEPRIL)
LOTENSIN HCT® (BENAZEPRIL/HCTZ)

Lotensin® is an ACE inhibitor used to treat patients with high blood pressure. Lotensin HCT® is a combination tablet that has Lotensin® plus a diuretic. A typical dose of Lotensin® is 20 mg daily, and the price of thirty tablets is $33.79. The price of Lotensin HCT® 20/25 mg is also $33.49. The annual cost of Lotensin® or Lotensin HCT, is about $400. To decrease your cost, consider the following alternatives:

1. Ask your doctor for samples.
2. Purchase larger quantities at a discount pharmacy such as those listed in Strategy 2.
3. Investigate the government programs listed in Strategy 6, including Medicaid, the Veterans Health Administration, and state assistance programs.
4. Ask your doctor if you may purchase 40 mg tablets of Lotensin® and use a pill cutter to slice the tablet into two 20 mg parts. Lotensin HCT® may also be sliced with your doctor's approval.
5. Ask your doctor if you may substitute generic benzepril as benazepril/HCTZ for brand-name Lotensin® or Lotensin HCT®.
6. Ask your doctor if you may substitute generic captopril, enalapril, or lisinopril for brand-name Lotensin®. These generic medications are also ACE inhibitors with similar indications. With your doctor's approval, take a generic diuretic and a generic ACE inhibitor instead of Lotensin HCT®.
7. Contact the Novartis Patient Assistance Program by telephoning 800-277-2254.

LOTREL® (AMLODIPINE/BENAZEPRIL)

Lotrel® is a combination tablet used to treat patients with high blood pressure containing Norvasc® (amlodipine), a calcium channel blocker, and Lotensin® (benazepril), an ACE inhibitor. A typical dose of Lotrel® 5/20 mg daily, and the price of thirty capsules is $68.27. The annual cost of this dose is about $820. To decrease your cost, consider the following alternatives:

1. Ask your doctor for samples.
2. Purchase larger quantities at a discount pharmacy such as those listed in Strategy 2.
3. Investigate the government programs listed in Strategy 6, including Medicaid, the Veterans Health Administration, and state assistance programs.
4. Since Lotrel® contains a brand-name ACE inhibitor (Lotensin®) and a brand-name calcium channel blocker, there are two substitutions involved. First, ask your doctor if you may substitute generic captopril, enalapril, or lisinopril for brand-name Lotensin®. These generic medications are also ACE inhibitors with similar indications. Ask your doctor if you may substitute a different calcium channel blocker such as generic Adalat®CC (extended-release nifedipine) for Norvase®. With your doctor's approval, take a generic calcium channel blocker and a generic ACE inhibitor instead of Lotrel®.
5. Contact the Novartis Patient Assistance Program by telephoning 800-277-2254.

LOVENOX® (ENOXAPARIN)

Lovenox® is a low molecular weight heparin used to thin the blood. A typical dose of Lovenox® to prevent harmful blood clot formation in those undergoing knee surgery is 30 mg injected subcutaneously twice daily for ten days. The price for twenty pre-filled 30 mg syringes is $367.74. To decrease your cost, consider the following alternatives:

1. Ask your doctor for samples.
2. Purchase larger quantities at a discount pharmacy such as those listed in Strategy 2.
3. Investigate the government programs listed in Strategy 6, including Medicaid, the Veterans Health Administration, and state assistance programs.
4. Contact the Lovenox Patient Assistance Program by having an advocate telephone 888-632-8607.

MAVIK® (TRANDOLAPRIL)
TARKA® (TRANDOLAPRIL/VERAPAMIL)

Mavik® is an ACE inhibitor used to treat patients with high blood pressure or congestive heart failure. Tarka® is a combination tablet that includes Mavik® and verapamil, a calcium channel blocker. A typical dose of Mavik® is 2 mg daily, and the price of thirty tablets is $36.39. The annual cost of Mavik® is about $430. The price of thirty tablets of a typical dose of Tarka® 2/180 mg is $63.59, and the annual cost of this dose is about $770. To decrease your cost, consider the following alternatives:

1. Ask your doctor for samples.
2. Purchase larger quantities at a discount pharmacy such as those listed in Strategy 2.
3. Investigate the government programs listed in Strategy 6, including Medicaid, the Veterans Health Administration, and state assistance programs.
4. Ask your doctor if you may purchase 4 mg tablets of Mavik® and use a pill cutter to slice the tablet into two 2 mg parts. Tarka® may also be sliced with your doctor's approval, although this is not usually done due to its dosage.
5. Ask your doctor if substituting generic captopril, enalapril, or lisinopril for brand-name Mavik® is appropriate. These generic medications are ACE inhibitors with similar indications. With your doctor's approval, take generic verapamil and a generic ACE inhibitor instead of Tarka®.
6. Contact the Abbott Laboratories Patient Assistance Program by having an advocate telephone 800-222-6885.

MICARDIS® (TELMISARTAN)
MICARDIS HCT® (TELMISARTAN/HCTZ)

Micardis® is an angiotensin receptor blocker used to treat patients with high blood pressure. Micardis HCT® is a combination tablet that contains Micardis® and a diuretic. A typical dose of Micardis® is 80mg daily, and the price of twenty-eight tablets is $48.99. The annual cost of this medication is about $590. The price of thirty tablets of a typical dose of Micardis HCT® 80/12.5 mg is $58.89, and the annual cost of this dose is $710. To decrease your cost, consider the following alternatives:

1. Ask your doctor for samples.
2. Purchase larger quantities at a discount pharmacy such as those listed in Strategy 2.
3. Investigate the government programs listed in Strategy 6, including Medicaid, the Veterans Health Administration, and state assistance programs.
4. Ask your doctor if you may purchase 80 mg tablets of Micardis® and use a pill cutter to slice the tablet into two 40 mg parts. Micardis HCT® may also be sliced with your doctor's approval.
5. Ask your doctor if you may substitute generic captopril, enalapril, or lisinopril for brand-name Micardis® These generic medications are ACE inhibitors and have similar indications to those of angiotensin receptor blockers. Some patients can't take ACE inhibitors because they develop a cough.
6. Ask your doctor if substituting a generic diuretic such as HCTZ or chlorthalidone and taking it with a generic ACE inhibitor is appropriate instead of taking Micardis HCT®.
7. Contact the Boehringer Ingelheim Care Foundation Patient Assistance Program by having an advocate telephone 800-556-8317.

MOBIC® (MELOXICAM)

Mobic® decreases inflammation by inhibiting the cyclooxygenase enzyme and is used to treat arthritis and muscle aches. A typical dose of Mobic® is 7.5 mg daily, and the price of thirty tablets is $85.37. Although it frequently is not taken on a daily basis for a year, the annual cost of this medication is about $1,025. To decrease your cost, consider the following alternatives:

1. Ask your doctor for samples.
2. Purchase larger quantities at a discount pharmacy such as those listed in Strategy 2.
3. Investigate the government programs listed in Strategy 6, including Medicaid, the Veterans Health Administration, and state assistance programs.
4. Ask your doctor if you may substitute a generic NSAID—such as ibuprofen or naproxen—for Mobic®. These medications are available without a prescription at much less cost.
5. Contact the Boehringer Ingelheim Care Foundation Patient Assistance Program by having an advocate telephone 800-556-8317.

MONOPRIL® (FOSINOPRIL)
MONOPRIL® HCT (FOSINOPRIL/HCTZ)

Monopril® is an ACE inhibitor used to treat patients with high blood pressure or congestive heart failure. Monopril HCT® is a combination tablet that has Monopril® and a diuretic within the tablet. A typical dose of Monopril® is 20 mg daily, and the price for thirty tablets is $39.09. The annual cost for this medication is about $470. A typical dose of Monopril HCT® is 20/12.5 mg, and the price for thirty tablets is generally similar to Monopril®. To decrease your cost, consider the following alternatives:

1. Ask your doctor for samples.
2. Purchase larger quantities at a discount pharmacy such as those listed in Strategy 2.
3. Investigate the government programs listed in Strategy 6, including Medicaid, the Veterans Health Administration, and state assistance programs.
4. Ask your doctor if you may purchase 40 mg tablets of Monopril® and use a pill cutter to slice the tablet into two 20 mg parts.
5. Ask your doctor if substituting generic fosinopril or fosinopril/HCTZ for brand-name Monopril® and Monopril HCT® is appropriate. Alternatively ask your doctor if substituting generic captopril, enalapril, or lisinopril for brand-name Monopril® is appropriate. These generic medications are also ACE inhibitors.
6. Ask your doctor if substituting a generic diuretic such as HCTZ or chlorthalidone and taking it with a generic ACE inhibitor instead of Monopril HCT® is appropriate.
7. Contact the Bristol-Myers Squibb Pharmaceutical Assistance Program by having an advocate telephone 800-736-0003.

NASONEX® (MOMETASONE)

Nasonex® is a nasal spray containing a corticosteroid used to treat patients with allergic rhinitis A typical dose for Nasonex® is two sprays in each nostril daily, and the price for one nasal pump mist bottle is $65.17. To decrease your cost, consider the following alternatives:

1. Ask your doctor for samples.
2. Purchase larger quantities at a discount pharmacy such as those listed in Strategy 2.
3. Investigate the government programs listed in Strategy 6, including Medicaid, the Veterans Health Administration, and state assistance programs.
4. Ask your doctor if over-the-counter, brand-name Afrin® (oxymetazoline) or its generic substitute is an appropriate substitute. These medications are not corticosteroids and provide relief from nasal congestion by a different mechanism.
5. Contact the GlaxoSmithKline Bridges to Access Program by having an advocate telephone 866-728-4368.

NEURONTIN® (GABAPENTIN)

Neurontin® is an analgesic used to manage pain. A typical dose of Neurontin® involves taking three 300 mg capsules daily, and the price of ninety tablets is about $120. The annual cost of this medication is about $1440. To decrease your cost, consider the following alternatives:

1. Ask your doctor for samples.
2. Purchase larger quantities at a discount pharmacy such as those listed in Strategy 2.
3. Investigate the government programs listed in Strategy 6, including Medicaid, the Veterans Health Administration, and state assistance programs.
4. Ask your doctor if you may purchase 600 mg tablets of Neurontin® and use a pill cutter to slice the tablet into two 300 mg parts. The 600 mg dose is available as a tablet, but the 300 mg dose is available as a capsule.
5. Ask your doctor if you may substitute generic gabapentin for brand-name Neurontin®.
6. Contact the Pfizer Connection to Care Program by having an advocate telephone 800-707-8990.

NEXIUM® (ESOMEPRAZOLE)

Nexium® is a proton pump inhibitor used to treat heartburn, ulcers, and acid reflux. A typical dose of Nexium® is 20 mg daily, and the price of thirty capsules is $123.07. Although it generally should not be taken on a daily basis for a year, the annual cost of this medication is about $1,470. To decrease your cost, consider the following alternatives:

1. Ask your doctor for samples.
2. Purchase larger quantities at a discount pharmacy such as those listed in Strategy 2.
3. Investigate the government programs listed in Strategy 6, including Medicaid, the Veterans Health Administration, and state assistance programs.
4. Ask your doctor if Prilosec® 20 mg daily would be an acceptable substitute for Nexium®. Prilosec® is available without a prescription at much less cost.
5. Ask your doctor if an H_2 blocker like generic cimetidine, ranitidine, or famotidine would be an acceptable substitute for Nexium®. These medications, which work differently than proton pump in hibitors, are available without a prescription at much less cost.
6. Contact the AstraZeneca Foundation Patient Assistance Program by having an advocate telephone 800-424-3727.

NOROXIN® (NORFLOXACIN)

Noroxin® is an antibiotic used to treat bacterial infections. A typical dose of Noroxin® is 400 mg tablets twice daily for seven days, and the price of seven tablets is about $55. To decrease your cost, consider the following alternatives:

1. Ask your doctor for samples.
2. Purchase larger quantities at a discount pharmacy such as those listed in Strategy 2.
3. Investigate the government programs listed in Strategy 6, including Medicaid, the Veterans Health Administration, and state assistance programs.
4. Ask your doctor if you may substitute generic ciprofloxacin for brand-name Noroxin®; both are quinolone antibiotics.
5. Ask your doctor if substituting a different type of antibiotic, such as generic amoxicillin or trimethoprim/sulfamethoxazole for brand-name Noroxin® is appropriate. Those who are allergic to penicillin cannot take amoxicillin and those who are allergic to sulfa cannot take trimethoprim/sulfamethoxazole.
6. Contact the Merck Patient Assistance Program by having an advocate telephone 800-944-2111.

NIASPAN® (EXTENDED-RELEASE NIACIN)

Niaspan® is a B vitamin with an unique extended-release formulation used to lower triglyceride and cholesterol levels. A typical dose of Niaspan® is 500 mg daily, and the price of thirty tablets is $46.29. The annual cost of this medication is about $550. To decrease your cost, consider the following alternatives:

1. Ask your doctor for samples.
2. Purchase larger quantities at a discount pharmacy such as those listed in Strategy 2.
3. Investigate the government programs listed in Strategy 6, including Medicaid, the Veterans Health Administration, and state assistance programs.
4. Ask your doctor if you may substitute generic SloNiacin® for Niaspan®. SloNiacin® is available without a prescription and is a different type of extended release niacin.
5. Contact the Kos Patient Assistance Program by having an advocate telephone 866-363-1024.

NORVASC® (AMLODIPINE)

Norvasc® is a calcium channel blocker used to treat patients with high blood pressure. A typical dose of Norvasc® is 5 mg daily, and the price of thirty tablets is $44.97. The annual cost of this medication is about $540. To decrease your cost, consider the following alternatives:

1. Ask your doctor for samples.
2. Purchase larger quantities at a discount pharmacy such as those listed in Strategy 2.
3. Investigate the government programs listed in Strategy 6, including Medicaid, the Veterans Health Administration, and state assistance programs.
4. Ask your doctor if you may purchase 10 mg tablets of Norvasc® and use a pill cutter to slice the tablet into two 5 mg parts.
5. Ask your doctor if substituting a different calcium channel blocker such as generic nifedipine or verapamil for brand-name Norvasc® is appropriate.
6. Ask your doctor if substituting a different type of blood pressure medication such as the generic diuretic, chlorthalidone, for brand-name Norvasc® is appropriate.
7. Contact the Pfizer Connection to Care Program by having an advocate telephone 800-707-8990.

ORTHO EVRA®
(NORELGESTROMIN/ETHINYL ESTRADIOL TRANSDERMAL SYSTEM)

Ortho Evra® is a contraceptive patch containing the female hormones estrogens and progestins. A typical monthly dose of Ortho Evra® involves applying a patch for three consecutive weeks beginning on the first day of your period. The fourth week is patch free. The price for a box of three patches is $37.99, and the annual cost is about $500. To decrease your cost, consider the following alternatives:

1. Ask your doctor for samples.
2. Purchase larger quantities at a discount pharmacy such as those listed in Strategy 2.
3. Investigate the government programs listed in Strategy 6, including Medicaid, the Veterans Health Administration, and state assistance programs.
4. Ask your doctor if taking a generic birth control pill, such as Necon®, Aviane®, or Apri®, would be an acceptable substitute. These generic birth control pills contain different hormones than Ortho Evra®.

ORTHO-NOVUM® (NORETHINDRONE/ETHINYL ESTRADIOL)

Ortho-Novum® is a contraceptive tablet containing estrogen and progestin. A typical dose of Ortho-Novum® is 1 mg/0.035 mg daily, and the price for twenty-eight tablets is $42.39. The annual cost for this medication is about $550. To decrease your cost, consider the following alternatives:

1. Ask your doctor for samples.
2. Purchase larger quantities at a discount pharmacy such as those listed in Strategy 2.
3. Investigate the government programs listed in Strategy 6, including Medicaid, the Veterans Health Administration, and state assistance programs.
4. Ask your doctor if taking Necon®, a generic version of Ortho-Novum®, would be an acceptable substitute for brand-name Ortho-Novum®.

ORTHO TRI-CYCLEN® (NORGESTIMATE/ESTRADIOL)

Ortho Tri-Cyclen® is a contraceptive tablet containing estrogen and progestin. A typical dose of Ortho Tri-Cyclen® is 0.25mg/0.035 mg daily, and the price for twenty-eight tablets is $36.99. The annual cost for this medication is about $480. To decrease your cost, consider the following alternatives:

1. Ask your doctor for samples.
2. Purchase larger quantities at a discount pharmacy such as those listed in Strategy 2.
3. Investigate the government programs listed in Strategy 6, including Medicaid, the Veterans Health Administration, and state assistance programs.
4. Ask your doctor if taking Tri-Nessa®, a generic version of Ortho Tri-Cyclen®, would be an acceptable substitute for brand-name Ortho Tri-Cyclen®.

PAXIL® (PAROXETINE)

Paxil® is a selective serotonin reuptake inhibitor, SSRI, antidepressant used to treat patients with major depression. A typical dose of Paxil® is 20 mg daily, and the price for thirty tablets is $81.49. The annual cost for this medication is about $980. Paxil XL™ is a controlled release version of Paxil®. To decrease your cost, consider the following alternatives:

1. Ask your doctor for samples.
2. Purchase larger quantities at a discount pharmacy such as those listed in Strategy 2.
3. Investigate the government programs listed in Strategy 6, including Medicaid, the Veterans Health Administration, and state assistance programs.
4. Purchase 40 mg tablets of Paxil® and use a pill cutter to slice the tablet into two 20 mg parts *if your doctor feels this is appropriate.*
5. Ask your doctor if you may substitute generic paroxetine for brand-name Paxil®.
6. Contact the GlaxoSmithKline Pharmaceutical Assistance Program by having an advocate telephone 866-728-4368.

PLAVIX® (CLOPIDOGREL)

Plavix® is a platelet inhibitor used to treat patients who recently had coronary angioplasty with stent placement. A typical dose of Plavix® is 75 mg once daily, and the price for thirty tablets is $116.27. The annual cost for this medication is about $1,400. To decrease your cost, consider the following alternatives:

1. Ask your doctor for samples.
2. Purchase larger quantities at a discount pharmacy such as those listed in Strategy 2.
3. Investigate the government programs listed in Strategy 6, including Medicaid, the Veterans Health Administration, and state assistance programs.
4. Contact the Bristol-Myers Squibb Pharmaceutical Assistance Foundation by having an advocate telephone 800-736-0003.

PLENDIL® (FELODIPINE)

Plendil® is a calcium channel blocker used to treat patients with high blood pressure. A typical dose of Plendil® is 5 mg daily, and the price of thirty tablets is $39.39. The annual cost of this medication is about $470. To decrease your cost, consider the following alternatives:

1. Ask your doctor for samples.
2. Purchase larger quantities at a discount pharmacy such as those listed in Strategy 2.
3. Investigate the government programs listed in Strategy 6, including Medicaid, the Veterans Health Administration, and state assistance programs.
4. Ask your doctor if you may substitute generic felodipine for brand-name Plendil®.
5. Ask your doctor if substituting a different calcium channel blocker such as generic nifedipine or verapamil for brand-name Plendil® is appropriate.
6. Contact the AstraZeneca Foundation Patient Assistance Program by having an advocate telephone 800-424-3727.

PLETAL® (CILOSTAZOL)

Pletal® is a phosphodiesterase III inhibitor used to treat claudication. A typical dose of Pletal® is 100 mg twice daily, and the price for sixty tablets is $115.42. The annual cost for this medication is about $1,380. To decrease your cost, consider the following alternatives:

1. Ask your doctor for samples.
2. Purchase larger quantities at a discount pharmacy such as those listed in Strategy 2.
3. Investigate the government programs listed in Strategy 6, including Medicaid, the Veterans Health Administration, and state assistance programs.
4. Ask your doctor if you may substitute generic cilostazol for brand-name Pletal®.
5. Ask your doctor if substituting generic pentoxifylline (Trental®) for brand-name Pletal® is appropriate. Trental® works by a different mechanism and may not be an appropriate substitute.
6. Contact the Patient Assistance Program for Pletal® by having an advocate telephone 800-992-4546.

PRAVACHOL® (PRAVASTATIN)

Pravachol® is a statin used to lower cholesterol levels, particularly the LDL cholesterol that clogs arteries. A typical dose of Pravachol® is 40 mg daily, and the price of thirty tablets is $127.77. The annual cost of this medication is about $1,530. To decrease your cost, consider the following alternatives:

1. Ask your doctor for samples.
2. Purchase larger quantities at a discount pharmacy such as those listed in Strategy 2.
3. Investigate the government programs listed in Strategy 6, including Medicaid, the Veterans Health Administration, and state assistance programs.
4. Ask your doctor if you may purchase 80 mg tablets of Pravachol® and use a pill cutter to slice the tablet into two 40 mg parts.
5. Ask your doctor if generic lovastatin would be an acceptable substitute for Pravachol®. The generic lovastatin may be sliced into two parts.
6. Ask your doctor if a sliced tablet of the more potent Lipitor® or Crestor® would be an acceptable substitute.
7. Contact the Bristol-Myers Squibb Patient Assistance Foundation by having an advocate telephone 800-736-0003.

PREMARIN® (CONJUGATED ESTROGENS)

Premarin® contains estrogen hormones used to treat women with menopausal symptoms. A typical dose of Premarin® is 0.625 mg daily, and the price for thirty tablets is $30.47. The annual cost for this medication is about $360. To decrease your cost, consider the following alternatives:

1. Ask your doctor for samples.
2. Purchase larger quantities at a discount pharmacy such as those listed in Strategy 2.
3. Investigate the government programs listed in Strategy 6, including Medicaid, the Veterans Health Administration, and state assistance programs..
4. Ask your doctor if taking a different type of generic estrogen medication, such as generic Estrace® (estradiol), would be an acceptable substitute for brand-name Premarin®.
5. Contact the Wyeth Pharmaceutical Assistance Program by having an advocate telephone 800-568-9938.

PREMPRO™ (CONJUGATED ESTROGENS/MEDROXYPROGESTERONE)

Prempro™ is a combination tablet containing estrogen and progestin hormones, and it is used to treat women with menopausal symptoms. A typical dose of Prempro™ is 0.45mg/1.5 mg daily, and the price for twenty eight tablets is $38.57. The annual cost for this medication is about $460. To decrease your cost, consider the following alternatives:

1. Ask your doctor for samples.
2. Purchase larger quantities at a discount pharmacy such as those listed in Strategy 2.
3. Investigate the government programs listed in Strategy 6, including Medicaid, the Veterans Health Administration, and state assistance programs.
4. Ask your doctor if taking a different type of generic estrogen, such as generic Estrace® (estradiol), and a generic progestin, such as Provera® (medroxyprogesterone), would be an acceptable substitute for brand name Prempro™.
5. Contact the Wyeth Pharmaceutical Assistance Program by having an advocate telephone 800-568-9938.

PREVACID® (LANSOPRAZOLE)

Prevacid® is a proton pump inhibitor used to treat heartburn, ulcers, and acid reflux. A typical dose of Prevacid® is 30 mg daily, and the price of thirty capsules is $123.07. Although it generally should not be taken on a daily basis for a year, the annual cost of this medication is about $1,480. To decrease your cost, consider the following alternatives:

1. Ask your doctor for samples.
2. Purchase larger quantities at a discount pharmacy such as those listed in Strategy 2.
3. Investigate the government programs listed in Strategy 6, including Medicaid, the Veterans Health Administration, and state assistance programs.
4. Ask your doctor if Prilosec® 20 mg daily would be an acceptable substitute for Prevacid®. Prilosec® is available without a prescription at much less cost.
5. Ask your doctor if an H_2 blocker like generic cimetidine, ranitidine, or famotidine would be an acceptable substitute for Prevacid®. These medications, which work differently than proton pump inhibitors, are available without a prescription at much less cost.
6. Contact the Prevacid Patient Assistance Program by having an advocate telephone 800-830-1015, option 1.

PRINIVIL® (LISINOPRIL)
PRINZIDE® (LISINOPRIL/HCTZ)

Prinivil® is an ACE inhibitor used to treat patients with high blood pressure or congestive heart failure. Prinzide® is a combination tablet that has Prinivil® and a diuretic within the tablet. A typical dose of Prinivil® is 20 mg daily, and the price for thirty tablets is $31.77. The annual cost for this medication is about $380. A typical dose of Prinzide® is 20/12.5 mg, and the price for thirty tablets is $37.19 for an annual cost of $450. To decrease your cost, consider the following alternatives:

1. Ask your doctor for samples.
2. Purchase larger quantities at a discount pharmacy such as those listed in Strategy 2.
3. Investigate the government programs listed in Strategy 6, including Medicaid, the Veterans Health Administration, and state assistance programs.
4. Ask your doctor if you may purchase 40 mg tablets of Prinivil® and use a pill cutter to slice the tablet into two 20 mg parts.
5. Ask your doctor if you may substitute generic lisinopril or lisinopril/HCTZ for brand name Prinivil® and Prinzide®.
6. Ask your doctor if substituting a generic diuretic such as HCTZ or chlorthalidone and taking it with generic lisinopril instead of Prinzide® is appropriate.
7. Contact the Merck Patient Assistance Program by having an advocate telephone 800-727-5400.

PROTONIX® (PANTOPRAZOLE)

Protonix® is a proton pump inhibitor used to treat heartburn, ulcers, and acid reflux. A typical dose of Protonix® is 20 mg daily, and the price of thirty tablets is $100.27. Although it generally should not be taken on a daily basis for a year, the annual cost of this medication is about $1,200. To decrease your cost, consider the following alternatives:

1. Ask your doctor for samples.
2. Purchase larger quantities at a discount pharmacy such as those listed in Strategy 2.
3. Investigate the government programs listed in Strategy 6, including Medicaid, the Veterans Health Administration, and state assistance programs.
4. Ask your doctor if Prilosec® 20 mg daily would be an acceptable substitute for Protonix®. Prilosec® is available without a prescription at much less cost.
5. Ask your doctor if an H_2 blocker like generic cimetidine, ranitidine, or famotidine would be an acceptable substitute for Protonix®. These medications, which work differently than proton pump inhibitors, are available without a prescription at much less cost.
6. Contact the Wyeth Pharmaceutical Assistance Foundation by having an advocate telephone 800-568-9938.

PROZAC® (FLUOXETINE)

Prozac® is a selective serotonin reuptake inhibitor, SSRI, antidepressant used to treat patients with major depression. A typical dose of Prozac® is 20 mg daily, and the price for thirty tablets is $114.39. The annual cost for this medication is about $1370. To decrease your cost, consider the following alternatives:

1. Ask your doctor for samples.
2. Purchase larger quantities at a discount pharmacy such as those listed in Strategy 2.
3. Investigate the government programs listed in Strategy 6, including Medicaid, the Veterans Health Administration, and state assistance programs.
4. Ask your doctor if substituting generic fluoxetine for brand-name Prozac® is appropriate.
5. Contact the Lilly Cares Patient Assistance Program by having an advocate telephone 800-545-6962.

REMERON® (MIRTAZAPINE)

Remeron® is a tetracyclic antidepressant used to treat patients with major depression. A typical dose of Remeron® is 30 mg daily, and the price of thirty tablets is $91.59. The annual cost of this medication is about $1,100. To decrease your cost, consider the following alternatives:

1. Ask your doctor for samples.
2. Purchase larger quantities at a discount pharmacy such as those listed in Strategy 2.
3. Investigate the government programs listed in Strategy 6, including Medicaid, the Veterans Health Administration, and state assistance programs.
4. Ask your doctor if you may purchase 45 mg tablets of Remeron® and use a pill cutter to slice the tablet into two 22.5 mg parts *if your doctor feels this is appropriate*. The 45 mg tablets are scored to facilitate slicing.
5. Ask your doctor if you may substitute generic mirtazapine for brand-name Remeron®.
6. Contact the Organon Pharmaceutical Assistance Program by having an advocate telephone 973-325-5273.

RISPERDAL® (RISPERIDONE)

Risperdal® is a powerful benzisoxazole derivative antipsychotic medication used to treat schizophrenia. A typical dose of Risperdal® is 2 mg twice daily, and the price for sixty tablets is about $320. The annual cost for this medication is about $3,840. To decrease your cost, consider the following alternatives:

1. Ask your doctor for samples.
2. Purchase at a discount pharmacy such as those listed in Strategy 2.
3. Investigate the government programs listed in Strategy 6, including Medicaid, the Veterans Health Administration, and state assistance programs.
4. Contact the Risperdal® Patient Assistance Program and Reimbursement Support Program by having an advocate telephone 800-652-6227, ext. 1.

SEROQUEL® (QUETIAPINE)

Seroquel® is a powerful dibenzothiazepine derivative antipsychotic medication used to treat schizophrenia. A typical dose of Seroquel® is 200mg twice daily, and the price for sixty tablets is about $330. The annual cost for this medication is about $3,960. To decrease your cost, consider the following alternatives:

1. Ask your doctor for samples.
2. Purchase at a discount pharmacy such as those listed in Strategy 2.
3. Investigate the government programs listed in Strategy 6, including Medicaid, the Veterans Health Administration, and state assistance programs.
4. Contact the AstraZeneca Foundation Patient Assistance Program by having an advocate telephone 800-424-3727.

SINGULAIR® (MONTELUKAST)

Singulair® is a leukotriene receptor blocker used to treat patients with asthma. A typical dose for Singulair® is 10 mg daily, and the price for thirty tablets is $86.89. The annual cost for this medication is about $1,040. To decrease your cost, consider the following alternatives:

1. Ask your doctor for samples.
2. Purchase larger quantities at a discount pharmacy such as those listed in Strategy 2.
3. Investigate the government programs listed in Strategy 6, including Medicaid, the Veterans Health Administration, and state assistance programs.
4. Contact the Merck Patient Assistance Program by having an advocate telephone 800-727-5400.

SYNTHROID® (LEVOTHYROXINE)

Synthroid® is a type of thyroid hormone given to treat patients with hypothyroidism, low thyroid levels. A typical dose of Synthroid® is 100 mcg daily, and the price for thirty tablets is $16.09. The annual cost for this medication is about $200. To decrease your cost, consider the following alternatives:

1. Ask your doctor for samples.
2. Purchase larger quantities at a discount pharmacy such as those listed in Strategy 2.
3. Investigate the government programs listed in Strategy 6, including Medicaid, the Veterans Health Administration, and state assistance programs.
4. Ask your doctor if taking generic levothyroxine would be an acceptable substitute for brand name Synthroid®.
5. Contact the Abbott Pharmaceutical Assistance Program by having an advocate telephone 800-222-6885.

TEQUIN® (GATIFLOXACIN)

Tequin® is an antibiotic used to treat bacterial infections. A typical dose of Tequin® is 400 mg tablets once daily for five days, and the price of five tablets is about $40. To decrease your cost, consider the following alternatives:

1. Ask your doctor for samples.
2. Purchase larger quantities at a discount pharmacy such as those listed in Strategy 2.
3. Investigate the government programs listed in Strategy 6, including Medicaid, the Veterans Health Administration, and state assistance programs.
4. Ask your doctor if you may substitute generic ciprofloxacin for brand-name Tequin®; both are quinolone antibiotics.
5. Ask your doctor if substituting a different type of antibiotic, such as generic amoxicillin or trimethoprim/sulfamethoxazole for brand-name Tequin® is appropriate. Those who are allergic to penicillin cannot take amoxicillin and those who are allergic to sulfa cannot take trimethoprim/sulfamethoxazole.
6. Contact the Bristol-Myers Squibb Patient Assistance Foundation by having an advocate telephone 800-736-0003.

TEVETEN® (EPROSARTAN)
TEVETEN HCT® (EPROSARTAN/HCTZ)

Teveten® is an angiotensin receptor blocker used to treat patients with high blood pressure. Teveten HCT® is a combination tablet that contains Teveten® and a diuretic. A typical dose of Teveten® is 600 mg daily, and the price of thirty tablets is $46.39. The annual cost of this medication is about $570. Surprisingly, there is no extra charge for the diuretic, so the price of thirty tablets of a typical dose of Teveten HCT® 600/12.5 mg is identical. To decrease your cost, consider the following alternatives:

1. Ask your doctor for samples.
2. Purchase larger quantities at a discount pharmacy such as those listed in Strategy 2.
3. Investigate the government programs listed in Strategy 6, including Medicaid, the Veterans Health Administration, and state assistance programs.
4. If you need a lower dose of Teveten® than 600 mg, ask your doctor if you may purchase 600 mg tablets of Teveten® and use a pill cutter to slice the tablet into two 300 mg parts. Teveten HCT® may also be sliced with your doctor's approval. These medications are uncommonly sliced due to their dosages.
5. Ask your doctor if you may substitute generic captopril, enalapril, or lisinopril for brand-name Teveten® is appropriate. These generic medications are ACE inhibitors and have similar indications to angiotensin receptor blockers. Some patients can't take ACE inhibitors because they develop a cough.
6. Ask your doctor if substituting a generic diuretic such as HCTZ or chlorthalidone and taking it with a generic ACE inhibitor instead of Teveten HCT® is appropriate.
7. Contact the Biovail Pharmaceuticals Patient Assistance Program by having an advocate telephone 800-268-7325.

TOPROL-XL® (METOPROLOL SUCCINATE)

Toprol-XL® is a beta-blocker used to treat patients with high blood pressure. A typical dose of Toprol-XL® is 50 mg once daily, and the price of a one-month supply of thirty tablets is about $24.37. The annual cost of this medication is about $300. To decrease your cost, consider the following alternatives:

1. Ask your doctor for samples.
2. Purchase larger quantities at a discount pharmacy such as those listed in Strategy 2.
3. Investigate the government programs listed in Strategy 6, including Medicaid, the Veterans Health Administration, and state assistance programs.
4. Ask your doctor if you may purchase 100 mg tablets of Toprol-XL® and use a pill cutter to slice the tablet into two 50 mg parts.
5. Ask your doctor if you may substitute generic Lopressor® (metoprolol tartrate) for Toprol-XL®. Generic metoprolol tartrate is also suitable for slicing if you doctor approves.
6. Contact the AstraZeneca Foundation Patient Assistance Program by having an advocate telephone 800-424-3727.

TRICOR® (FENOFIBRATE)

Tricor® is a fibric acid derivative used to lower triglyceride levels. A typical dose of Tricor® is 145 mg daily, and the price of thirty tablets is $91.29. The annual cost of this medication is about $1,100. To decrease your cost, consider the following alternatives:

1. Ask your doctor for samples.
2. Purchase larger quantities at a discount pharmacy such as those listed in Strategy 2.
3. Investigate the government programs listed in Strategy 6, including Medicaid, the Veterans Health Administration, and state assistance programs.
4. Ask your doctor if you may substitute generic gemfibrozil or Slo-Niacin® for Tricor®. Generic gemfibrozil is a fibric acid derivative and lowers triglycerides by a mechanism similar to fenofibrate. SloNiacin® lowers triglycerides by a different mechanism.
5. Contact the Abbott Laboratories Patient Assistance Program by having an advocate telephone 800-222-6885.

VALTREX® (VALACYCLOVIR)

Valtrex® is an antiviral medication used to treat Herpes infections. A typical dose of Valtrex® used to treat Herpes Zoster infections is 1 gram every eight hours for seven days. The price for thirty tablets is $249.49. To decrease your cost, consider the following alternatives:

1. Ask your doctor for samples.
2. Purchase larger quantities at a discount pharmacy such as those listed in Strategy 2.
3. Investigate the government programs listed in Strategy 6, including Medicaid, the Veterans Health Administration, and state assistance programs.
4. Contact the GlaxoSmithKline Bridges to Access Program by having an advocate telephone 866-728-4368.

VIAGRA® (SILDENAFIL)

Viagra® is used to treat patients with erectile dysfunction. A typical dose of Viagra® is 50 mg, and the price of thirty tablets is $273.64. To decrease your cost, consider the following alternatives:

1. Ask your doctor for samples.
2. Purchase larger quantities at a discount pharmacy such as those listed in Strategy 2.
3. Investigate the government programs listed in Strategy 6, including Medicaid, the Veterans Health Administration, and state assistance programs.
4. Ask your doctor if you may purchase 100 mg tablets of Viagra® and use a pill cutter to slice the tablet into two 50 mg parts.
5. Contact the Pfizer Connection to Care Program by having an advocate telephone 800-707-8990.

WELLBUTRIN SR® (BUPROPION)

Wellbutrin SR® is an aminoketone antidepressant used to treat patients with major depression. A typical dose of Wellbutrin SR® 150 mg daily, and the price of thirty tablets is $61.79. The annual cost of this medication is about $740. To decrease your cost, consider the following alternatives:

1. Ask your doctor for samples.
2. Purchase larger quantities at a discount pharmacy such as those listed in Strategy 2.
3. Investigate the government programs listed in Strategy 6, including Medicaid, the Veterans Health Administration, and state assistance programs.
4. Ask your doctor if substituting generic bupropion for brand-name Wellbutrin SR® is appropriate.
5. Contact the GlaxoSmithKline Bridges to Access Program by having an advocate telephone 866-728-4368.

ZESTRIL® (LISINOPRIL)
ZESTORETIC® (LISINOPRIL/HCTZ)

Zestril® is an ACE inhibitor used to treat patients with high blood pressure or congestive heart failure. Zestoretic® is a combination tablet that has Zestril® and a diuretic within the tablet. A typical dose of Zestril® is 20 mg daily, and the price for thirty tablets is $35.39. The annual cost for this medication is about $425. A typical dose of Zestoretic® is 20/12.5 mg, and the price for thirty tablets is $40.27 for an annual cost of $480. To decrease your cost, consider the following alternatives:

1. Ask your doctor for samples.
2. Purchase larger quantities at a discount pharmacy such as those listed in Strategy 2.
3. Investigate the government programs listed in Strategy 6, including Medicaid, the Veterans Health Administration, and state assistance programs.
4. Ask your doctor if you may purchase 40 mg tablets of Zestril® and use a pill cutter to slice the tablet into two 20 mg parts.
5. Ask your doctor if you may substitute generic lisinopril or lisinopril/HCTZ for brand name Zestril® and Zestoretic® is appropriate.
6. Ask your doctor if substituting a generic diuretic such as HCTZ or chlorthalidone and taking it with generic lisinopril instead of Zestoretic® is appropriate.

ZIAC® (BISOPROLOL/HCTZ)

Ziac® is a combination tablet used to treat patients with high blood pressure. Ziac® contains both a beta-blocker, Zebeta® (bisoprolol), and a diuretic, HCTZ. A typical dose of Ziac® is 2.5/6.25 mg daily, and the price of thirty tablets is $47.39. The annual cost of this medication is about $570. To decrease your cost, consider the following alternatives:

1. Ask your doctor for samples.
2. Purchase larger quantities at a discount pharmacy such as those listed in Strategy 2.
3. Investigate the government programs listed in Strategy 6, including Medicaid, the Veterans Health Administration, and state assistance programs.
4. Substitute generic bisoprolol/HCTZ for Ziac®.
5. Ask your doctor if you may take a generic diuretic such as HCTZ or chlorthalidone with a generic beta-blocker such as atenolol or metoprolol tartrate instead of Ziac®.
6. Contact the Wyeth Pharmaceutical Assistance Foundation by having an advocate telephone 800-568-9938.

ZITHROMAX® (AZITHROMYCIN)

Zithromax® is an antibiotic frequently used to treat bacterial infections. A typical dose of Zithromax® involves taking two 250 mg tablets on the first day then taking one tablet daily for four days, and the price of six tablets is $47.99. To decrease your cost, consider the following alternatives:

1. Ask your doctor for samples.
2. Purchase at a discount pharmacy such as those listed in Strategy 2.
3. Investigate the government programs listed in Strategy 6, including Medicaid, the Veterans Health Administration, and state assistance programs.
4. Ask your doctor if taking a different type of antibiotic, such as generic amoxicillin, for brand-name Zithromax® is appropriate. Those who are allergic to penicillin cannot take amoxicillin.
5. Contact the Pfizer Connection to Care Program by having an advocate telephone 800-707-8990.

ZOCOR® (SIMVASTATIN)

Zocor® is a statin used to lower cholesterol levels, particularly the LDL cholesterol that clogs arteries. A typical dose of Zocor® is 40 mg daily, and the price of thirty tablets is $127.87. The annual cost of this medication is about $1,530. To decrease your cost, consider the following alternatives:

1. Ask your doctor for samples.
2. Purchase larger quantities at a discount pharmacy such as those listed in Strategy 2.
3. Investigate the government programs listed in Strategy 6, including Medicaid, the Veterans Health Administration, and state assistance programs.
4. Ask your doctor if you may purchase 80 mg tablets of Zocor® and use a pill cutter to slice the tablet into two 40 mg parts.
5. Ask your doctor if you may substitute generic lovastatin for Zocor®. The generic lovastatin may be sliced into two parts.
6. Ask your doctor if a sliced tablet of the more potent Lipitor® or Crestor® would be an acceptable substitute. Both of these medications may be sliced into two parts.
7. Contact the Merck Patient Assistance Program by having an advocate telephone 800-727-5400.

ZOFRAN® (ONDANSETRON)

Zofran® is used to treat and prevent nausea and vomiting. A typical dose of Zofran® is 4 mg as needed, and the price of thirty tablets is $625.09. To decrease your cost, consider the following alternatives:

1. Ask your doctor for samples.
2. Purchase larger quantities at a discount pharmacy such as those listed in Strategy 2.
3. Investigate the government programs listed in Strategy 6, including Medicaid, the Veterans Health Administration, and state assistance programs.
4. Ask your doctor if a different medication such as Phenergan® (promethazine) or Compazine® (prochlorperazine) is an appropriate substitute.
5. Contact the GlaxoSmithKline Bridges to Access Program by having an advocate telephone 866-728-4368.

ZOLOFT® (SERTRALINE)

Zoloft® is a selective serotonin reuptake inhibitor (SSRI) antidepressant used to treat patients with major depression. A typical dose of Zoloft® is 50 mg daily, and the price of thirty tablets is $76.57. The annual cost of this medication is about $920. To decrease your cost, you could consider the following alternatives.

1. Ask your doctor for samples.
2. Purchase larger quantities at a discount pharmacy such as those listed in Strategy 2.
3. Investigate the government programs listed in Strategy 6, including Medicaid, the Veterans Health Administration, and state assistance programs.
4. Purchase 100 mg tablets of Zoloft and use a pill cutter to slice the tablet into two 50 mg parts *if your doctor feels this is appropriate.*
5. Contact the Pfizer Connection to Care Program by having an advocate telephone 800-707-8990.

ZOVIRAX® (ACYCLOVIR)

Zovirax® is an antiviral medication used to treat Herpes infections. A typical dose of Zovirax® used to treat Herpes Zoster infections involves taking 800 mg five times daily for seven to ten days. The price for fifty tablets is $310.19. To decrease your cost, consider the following alternatives:

1. Ask your doctor for samples.
2. Purchase larger quantities at a discount pharmacy such as those listed in Strategy 2.
3. Investigate the government programs listed in Strategy 6, including Medicaid, the Veterans Health Administration, and state assistance programs.
4. Substitute generic acyclovir for brand-name Zovirax®.
5. Contact the GlaxoSmithKline Bridges to Access Program by having an advocate telephone 866-728-4368.

ZYPREXA® (OLANZAPINE)

Zyprexa® is a powerful thienobenzodiazepine antipsychotic medication used to treat schizophrenia. A typical dose of Zyprexa® is 10 mg daily, and the price for thirty tablets is $291.69. The annual cost for this medication is about $3,500. To decrease your cost, consider the following alternatives:

1. Ask your doctor for samples.
2. Purchase at a discount pharmacy such as those listed in Strategy 2.
3. Investigate the government programs listed in Strategy 6, including Medicaid, the Veterans Health Administration, and state assistance programs.
4. Contact the Lilly Cares Patient Assistance Program by having an advocate telephone 800-545-6962.

ZYRTEC® (CETIRIZINE)
ZYRTEC-D® (CETIRIZINE/PSEUDOEPHEDRINE)

Zyrtec® is a nonsedating antihistamine used to treat seasonal allergy symptoms, including watery eyes and runny nose. Zyrtec-D® is an extended release combination tablet of Zyrtec® and pseudoephedrine, a decongestant available without prescription. A typical dose of Zyrtec® is 10 mg daily, and the price of thirty tablets is $60.19. Although it generally should not be taken on a daily basis for a year, the annual cost of this medication is about $720. A typical dose of Zyrtec-D® is 5 mg/120mg daily, and the price of thirty tablets is $33.89 with an annual cost of about $400. To decrease your cost, consider the following alternatives:

1. Ask your doctor for samples.
2. Purchase larger quantities at a discount pharmacy such as those listed in Strategy 2.
3. Investigate the government programs listed in Strategy 6, including Medicaid, the Veterans Health Administration, and state assistance programs.
4. Ask your doctor if Claritin® or generic loratadine 10 mg daily would be an acceptable substitute for Zyrtec®. Both Claritin® and generic loratadine are available without a prescription at much less cost.
5. Ask your doctor if substituting over-the-counter pseudoephedrine and Zyrtec® or over-the-counter loratadine and pseudoephedrine for Zyrtec-D® is appropriate. Because pseudoephedrine is an ingredient in the illegal manufacturing of methamphetamine, sales of this medication may be limited.
6. Contact the Pfizer Connection to Care Program by having an advocate telephone 800-707-8990.

Appendix A: Websites and Additional Resources

Information on the Process of Drug Manufacturing and Distribution

Center for Drug Evaluation and Research (U.S. Food and Drug Administration)
www.fda.gov/cder/ogd/index.htm
Explains the process of generic drug approval.

"Report to the President: Prescription Drug Coverage, Spending, Utilization, and Prices" (Department of Health and Human Services, April 2000)
http://aspe.hhs.gov/health/reports/drugstudy/
Explains how pharmaceuticals travel from manufacturing plants, to retail pharmacies, then to consumers, and who pays for what along the way.

"How New Drugs Move Through the Development and Approval Process" (Tufts Center for the Study of Drug Development, November 2001)
http://csdd.tufts.edu/NewsEvents/RecentNews.asp?newsid=4
Explains the process of developing new drugs.

Lists of Drug Prices

Federal Supply Schedule
www.vapbm.org/PBM/prices.htm
Lists prices available to Veterans Hospitals, the Department of Defense, the Coast Guard, the Public Health Service, Indian tribes, and a few other organizations; the FSS prices must be equal to or lower than the best price offered by the drug company to any other buyer under similar conditions.

Destination Rx™
www.destinationrx.com
Compares prices at various online pharmacies.

PharmacyChecker.com
www.pharmacychecker.com
Compares prices at various online, mostly foreign, pharmacies.

The Red Book (published by Thomson Corporation)
800-678-5689
Lists the average wholesale price (AWP) of drugs.

Information on Government Programs
Centers for Medicare & Medicaid Services
www.cms.hhs.gov
Information about Medicare and Medicaid.

Medicaid
www.cms.hhs.gov/medicaid/
Information about Medicaid, as well as links to individual states' programs.

Medicare
www.medicare.gov
800-MEDICARE (800-633-4227)
Information about Medicare and Medicare-approved discount cards.

Ryan White Comprehensive AIDS Resources Emergency (CARE) Act
http://hab.hrsa.gov/history.htm
Information about government-provided health care for those with
AIDS and HIV disease.

Department of Veterans Affairs
www.va.gov
866-472-8333
877-222-VETS
Information about health benefits available to veterans. Military
retirees can call the Department of Defense at 800-538-9552.

Information on Discount Drug Programs

I-SaveRx
www.i-saverx.net
Assists Illinois, Wisconsin, Kansas, and Missouri residents to purchase
discounted pharmaceuticals from Canada, Ireland, and the United
Kingdom.

NeedyMeds
www.needymeds.com
Information on pharmaceutical companies' assistance programs.

Partnership for Prescription Assistance
www.pparx.org
888-471-2669
Offers a single point of access to more than 275 public and private
patient assistance programs, including more than 150 programs
offered by pharmaceutical companies.

Rx Outreach
www.rxoutreach.com
Express Scripts Specialty Distribution Services, Inc.
P.O. Box 66536
Saint Louis, MO 63166-6536
800-769-3880
Discount program for generic drugs.

Together Rx™
www.togetherrx.com
Information on a program that offers discounts to eligible Medicare recipients on drugs manufactured by a consortium of pharmaceutical companies, including Abbott, AstraZeneca, Aventis, Bristol-Myers Squibb, GlaxoSmithKline, Janssen, Novartis, and Ortho-McNeil.

Internet Pharmacies
Costco
www.costco.com/Pharmacy/FramMaster.asp?cat=678

Drugstore.com
www.drugstore.com

Family Meds
www.familymeds.com

General Information
American Association of Retired Persons
www.aarp.org
Lobbying group representing older persons.

Kaiser Family Foundation
www.kff.org
A nonprofit foundation focusing on the major health care issues facing the nation.

National Association of Boards of Pharmacy
www.nabp.net
847-391-4406
Lists licensed pharmacies in good standing.

Appendix B:
2005 Federal
Poverty Guidelines

Eligibility for many government assistance programs and pharmaceutical assistance programs are based on the Federal Poverty Guidelines. The 2004 Federal Poverty Guidelines were used throughout the book as they were most current. The 2005 Guidelines were published as the book was going to the printer and presented as a reference.

2005 Federal Poverty Guidelines			
NUMBER OF FAMILY MEMBERS IN HOUSEHOLD*	MAXIMUM INCOME IF LIVING IN THE LOWER 48 STATES OR WASHINGTON, D.C.	MAXIMUM INCOME IF LIVING IN ALASKA	MAXIMUM INCOME IF LIVING IN HAWAII
1	$9,570	$11,950	$11,010
2	$12,830	$16,030	$14,760
3	$16,090	$20,110	$18,510
4	$19,350	$24,190	$22,260
For each additional person, add	$3,260	$4,080	$3,750

* A household consists of all the persons who occupy a housing unit (house or apartment) whether they are related or not.

Appendix C:
Rx Outreach Application

Rx Outreach[SM]

Rx Outreach[SM] is a patient assistance program that provides more than 50 FDA-approved generic medicines to help you treat ongoing health problems. The program helps you get medicines you can afford. Rx Outreach provides a three-month supply of a medicine for $18. A six-month supply of a medicine costs $30.

Step 1: See if you qualify.
You can use Rx Outreach regardless of your age. You can use Rx Outreach even if you use another discount medicine program or patient assistance program. To use Rx Outreach, your income needs to be less than a certain amount of money each year. This amount varies depending on the number of financially dependent people living in your house.

Number of People in Your Household, Including Yourself*	All States and Washington D.C., Except Alaska and Hawaii	Alaska	Hawaii
You	Less than $23,275 a year	Less than $29,075 a year	Less than $26,750 a year
You + 1	Less than $31,225 a year	Less than $39,025 a year	Less than $35,900 a year
You + 2	Less than $39,175 a year	Less than $48,975 a year	Less than $45,050 a year
You + 3	Less than $47,125 a year	Less than $58,925 a year	Less than $54,200 a year
Add this amount for each additional person.*	$7,950 a year	$9,950 a year	$9,150 a year

Step 2: See if your medicines are included.
The list of medicines included in Rx Outreach can be found below.
Step 3: Call or visit your doctor for a prescription.

It is important that your doctor writes a prescription for a 90-day or 180-day supply of medicine.

Step 4: Find out how much money you need to send.
For each three-month (or 90-day) supply of medicine you order, you will pay $18. For each six-month (or 180-day) supply of medicine you order, you will pay $30. You can pay with checks, money orders, or credit cards (only Visa, MasterCard, or Discover). You need to send payment for the total amount. **Please do not send cash. If you have health insurance, you cannot use your insurance to help pay the fee for Rx Outreach.**

Step 5: Fill out and sign the Rx Outreach form.
Your medicine will be sent in a secure package to the address you give us – it can be your house, doctor's office, or trusted friend's house.

Step 6: Send in your payment, prescription, and form.
Send these three items in a stamped envelope to:

Rx Outreach
Express Scripts Specialty Distribution Services, Inc.
P.O. Box 66536
St. Louis, MO 63166-6536

If you have questions about your order, call us toll-free at 1-800-769-3880, Monday through Friday, 8:00 a.m. to 5:30 p.m. Central Time.

You can get the generic medicines listed below through Rx Outreach. The generic name of the medicine is listed first. The brand name is listed second. **Rx Outreach provides all strengths or doses of the medicines we carry.**

Arthritis and Gout
• Allopurinol tablet (Zyloprim®)
• Ibuprofen tablet (Motrin®)
• Naproxen tablet (Naprosyn®)

Asthma
• Albuterol tablet (Proventil®)
• Albuterol inhaler (Proventil®)

Bladder
• Oxybutynin tablet (Ditropan®)

Cancer
• Tamoxifen Citrate tablet (Nolvadex®)

Cholesterol, Triglycerides, Blood and Heart
• Digoxin tablet (Lanoxin®)
• Folic Acid tablet

• Gemfibrozil tablet (Lopid®)
• Lovastatin tablet (Mevacor®)
• Potassium Chloride ER tablet

Diabetes
• Glipizide tablet (Glucotrol®)
• Glipizide ER tablet (Glucotrol XL®)
• Glyburide tablet (DiaBeta® or Micronase®)
• Glyburide, micronized tablet (Glynase® PresTab®)
• Metformin HCL tablet (Glucophage®)
• Metformin HCL ER tablet (Glucophage XR®)

Diuretics and Blood Pressure
• Atenolol tablet (Tenormin®)
• Atenolol/Chlorthalidone tablet (Tenoretic®)
• Benazepril tablet (Lotensin®)
• Benazepril/HCTZ tablet (Lotensin HCT®)
• Bumetanide tablet (Bumex®)

• Captopril tablet (Capoten®)
• Clonidine HCL tablet (Catapres®)
• Doxazosin Mesylate tablet (Cardura®)
• Enalapril Maleate tablet (Vasotec®)
• Furosemide tablet (Lasix®)
• Hydrochlorothiazide tablet (Esidrix®, HydroDIURIL®)
• Hydrochlorothiazide capsule (Microzide®)
• Indapamide tablet (Lozol®)
• Labetalol HCL tablet (Trandate®)
• Lisinopril tablet (Zestril® or Prinivil®)
• Lisinopril/HCTZ tablet (Zestoretic® or Prinzide®)
• Metoprolol tablet (Lopressor®)
• Nadolol tablet (Corgard®)
• Propranolol tablet (Inderal®)
• Terazosin capsule (Hytrin®)
• Triamterene/HCTZ capsule (Dyazide®)
• Triamterene/HCTZ capsule

• Triamterene/HCTZ tablet (Maxzide®)
• Verapamil tablet (Calan® or Isoptin®)
• Verapamil SR tablet (Isoptin SR®)

Depression and Anxiety
• Amitriptyline tablet
• Buspirone tablet (BuSpar®)
• Fluoxetine capsule (Prozac®)
• Nortriptyline HCL capsule (Pamelor®)
• Trazodone tablet (Desyrel®)

Heartburn, Acid Reflux, Ulcers
• Famotidine tablet (Pepcid®)
• Metoclopramide HCL tablet (Reglan®)
• Omeprazole capsule (Prilosec®)
• Ranitidine tablet (Zantac®)

Hormones and Steroids
• Estradiol tablet (Estrace®)
• Prednisone tablet (Deltasone®)

Over

REV 9.04

About Your Doctor

Doctor's first name: _____ Doctor's last name: _____

Address: _____

City: _____ State: _____ ZIP code: _____

Phone number: (___) _____

If your doctor is helping you fill out this form, please ask that he or she tell us these three things. This information is not required for you to use Rx Outreach℠.

E-mail: _____ D.E.A. #: _____ State licensure #: _____

About You

First name: _____ Last name: _____

Date of birth: _____-_____-_____ Social Security # or green card #: _____

Address: _____

City: _____ State: _____ ZIP code: _____

Phone number: (___) _____

Male/Female: _____ E-mail: _____ *(optional)*

Please list any medicines you are allergic to: _____

Please list all medicines you are currently taking: _____

Shipping address if different from above:

Name: _____

Address: _____ City: _____ State: _____ ZIP code: _____

Income Information

Gross yearly income: _____ Number of people in your household, including yourself: _____

How to Pay

By check or money order: Please make payable to Rx Outreach.

By credit card: Include credit card number: ☐☐☐☐ ☐☐☐☐ ☐☐☐☐ ☐☐☐☐ Expiration date: ☐☐/☐☐

Check the type of credit card that you are using: ○ Visa ○ MasterCard ○ Discover

I authorize Express Scripts Specialty Distribution Services, Inc., to charge this credit card for payment.

Name on card: _____ Signature of cardholder: _____

# of 90-day prescriptions: _____ # of 180-day prescriptions: _____ Total payment enclosed: _____

You must sign the form before we can send you your medicines.
I attest that the information provided in this application is complete and accurate. This authorization or a copy shall be valid for 12 months from the date of signature. I understand that Express Scripts Speciality Distribution Services, Inc., reserves the right to refuse my application to the Rx Outreach Patient Assistance Program based on any misuse, abuse, or illegal distribution of any products in this program. I will not seek reimbursement of any fee I pay to Rx Outreach from my health insurance, including Medicaid, Medicare, or similar programs

| SIGN HERE | _____ Date: _____ / _____ / _____ |

138

Rx Outreach is managed by Express Scripts Specialty Distribution Services, Inc., (ESSDS), a fully licensed pharmacy. The company is committed to making the use of prescription drugs safer and more affordable. ESSDS reserves the right to add or delete medicines available in Rx Outreach, change fees in Rx Outreach, or discontinue Rx Outreach at any time. ESSDS does not accept returns of unused medicine, and fees are nonrefundable once ESSDS receives your prescription. ESSDS will send your medicines to the address you choose. You are responsible for the package once it arrives.

1-800-769-3880   *www.rxoutreach.com*

REV 9.04

Index

Note: All brand-name drugs are listed in **bold**. All generic drugs are listed in *italics*.